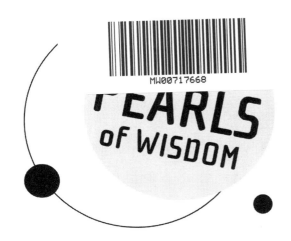

PEARLS
of WISDOM

The Poison Quiz Book

Second Edition

John Harris Trestrail III, *RPh, FAACT, DABAT*

McGraw-Hill
Medical Publishing Division

New York Chicago San Francisco Lisbon London
Madrid Mexico City Milan New Delhi
San Juan Seoul Singapore
Sydney Toronto

The Poison Quiz Book, Second Edition

Copyright © 2006 by The McGraw-Hill Companies, Inc. All rights reserved. Printed in the United States of America. Except as permitted under the United States Copyright Act of 1976, no part of this publication may be reproduced or distributed in any form or by any means, or stored in a data base or retrieval system, without the prior written permission of the publisher.

1 2 3 4 5 6 7 8 9 0   CUS/CUS   0 9 8 7 6 5

ISBN 0-07-146449-2

Notice

Medicine is an ever-changing science. As new research and clinical experience broaden our knowledge, changes in treatment and drug therapy are required. The authors and the publisher of this work have checked with sources believed to be reliable in their efforts to provide information that is complete and generally in accord with the standards accepted at the time of publication. However, in view of the possibility of human error or changes in medical sciences, neither the authors nor the publisher nor any other party who has been involved in the preparation or publication of this work warrants that the information contained herein is in every respect accurate or complete, and they disclaim all responsibility for any errors or omissions or for the results obtained from use of the information contained in this work. Readers are encouraged to confirm the information contained herein with other sources. For example and in particular, readers are advised to check the product information sheet included in the package of each drug they plan to administer to be certain that the information contained in this work is accurate and that changes have not been made in the recommended dose or in the contraindications for administration. This recommendation is of particular importance in connection with new or infrequently used drugs.

The editors were Catherine A. Johnson and Marsha Loeb.
The production supervisor was Phil Galea.
The cover designer was Handel Low.
Von Hoffmann Graphics was printer and binder.

This book is printed on acid-free paper.

Cataloging-in-Publication data for this title is on file at the Library of Congress.

DEDICATION

This book is dedicated to my parents, John Harris Trestrail and Edith (McClay) Trestrail, my wife Mary (Wenzel) Trestrail, our two children, John and Amanda, and our grandchildren, Olivia and Owen, without whose continued support and confidence, this labor of passion would not have been possible.

John

ABOUT THE AUTHOR

John Harris Trestrail III, *RPh, FAACT, DABAT*
Grand Rapids, Michigan

Mr. Trestrail graduated with honors, obtaining a B.S. degree in Pharmacy, from *Ferris State University*, Big Rapids, Michigan, in 1967, where he was initiated into *Rho Chi* (Pharmaceutical Honors Society). From 1967-1968, he attended graduate school, majoring in *natural product chemistry*, at the College of Pharmacy, *The Ohio State University*, Columbus, Ohio. Mr. Trestrail's public service experience was with the *United States Peace Corps*, from 1968-1970, where he taught chemistry at the *University of the Philippines College of Agriculture*, in the Republic of the Philippines. He is a practicing boarded toxicologist, and was a visiting instructor at the *FBI National Academy* in Quantico, Virginia. Since 1976, he has served as the Managing Director of one of the nation's certified regional poison centers.

He has been honored as a Fellow by the *American Academy of Clinical Toxicology*, and is a Diplomate, by examination, of the *American Board of Applied Toxicology*. Mr. Trestrail founded the *Center for the Study of Criminal Poisoning*, as well as the *Toxicological History Society*, and has been featured in several episodes of *"The New Detectives,"* on the *Discovery Channel*. He is a participant in the *International Program on Clinical Safety*, of the *World Health Organization (WHO)*. Mr. Trestrail has also served as an expert consultant in many criminal poisoning investigations, to law enforcement and attorneys. Since 1990, Mr Trestrail's seminars on *"Murder by Poison!"* and *"Poisoners Throughout History,"* have been received with wide acclaim by audiences throughout the United States, Canada, Europe, and Asia. He is the author of the pioneering book — *Criminal Poisoning: An Investigational Guide for Law Enforcement, Toxicologists, Forensic Scientists, and Attorneys*, published by *Humana Press*.

Since 1986, he has been the creator, producer, and moderator of the very popular *"Toxicology Quiz Bowl,"* sponsored annually by the **American Association of Poison Control Centers**, at the *North American Congress of Clinical Toxicology*. The majority of the questions found in this book, were compiled from actual toxicological trivia questions used in these annual competitions.

Mr. Trestrail is a member of the following professional organizations:

The American Academy of Clinical Toxicology (*AACT***)**
The American Association of Poison Control Centers (*AAPCC***)**
The American Academy of Forensic Sciences (*AAFS***)**
The International Homicide Investigators Association (*IHIA***)**
The North American Mycological Association (*NAMA***)**
The Society of Forensic Toxicology (*SOFT***)**

INTRODUCTION

Congratulations! *The Poison Quiz Book: Pearls of Wisdom*, will help you learn some medicine. Originally designed as a study aid to improve performance on the Inservice and Written Board exams, this book is full of useful information. A few words are appropriate discussing intent, format, limitations, and use.

Since this book is primarily intended as a study aid, the text is written in rapid-fire question/answer format. This way, readers receive immediate gratification. Moreover, misleading or confusing "foils" are not provided. This eliminates the risk of erroneously assimilating an incorrect piece of information that makes a big impression. Questions themselves often contain a "pearl" intended to reinforce the answer. Additional "hooks" may be attached to the answer in various forms, including mnemonics, visual imagery, repetition, and humor. Additional information not requested in the question may be included in the answer. Emphasis has been placed on distilling trivia and key facts that are easily overlooked, that are quickly forgotten, and that somehow seem to be needed on board examinations.

Many questions have answers without explanations. This enhances ease of reading and rate of learning. Explanations often occur in a later question/answer. Upon reading an answer, the reader may think, "Hm, why is that?" or, "Are you sure?" If this happens to you, go check! Truly assimilating these disparate facts into a framework of knowledge absolutely requires further reading of the surrounding concepts. Information learned in response to seeking an answer to a particular question is retained much better than information that is passively observed. Take advantage of this! Use this book with your preferred source texts handy and open.

The first half of the text is presented in topic areas found on the Inservice and Board Examination. The second section of the book, "Medicine Pearls," consists of medical topics often found on the inservice and board exam.

The Poison Quiz Book has limitations. We have found many conflicts between sources of information. We have tried to verify in several references the most accurate information. Some texts have internal discrepancies further confounding clarification.

The Poison Quiz Book risks accuracy by aggressively pruning complex concepts down to the simplest kernel—the dynamic knowledge base and clinical practice of medicine is not like that! Furthermore, new research and practice occasionally deviates from that which likely represents the right answer for test purposes. This text is designed to maximize your score on a test. Refer to your most current sources of information and mentors for direction.

The Poison Quiz Book is designed to be used, not just read. It is an *interactive* text. Use a 3 x 5 card and cover the answers; attempt all questions. A study method we recommend is oral, group study, preferably over an extended meal or pitchers. The mechanics of this method are simple and no one ever appears stupid. One person holds the book, with answers covered, and reads the question. Each person, including the reader, says "Check!" when he or she has an answer in mind. After everyone has "checked" in, someone states his/her answer. If this answer is correct, on to the next one; if not, another person says their answer or the answer can be read. Usually the person who "checks" in first receives the first shot at stating the answer. If this person is being a smarty-pants answer-hog, then others can take turns. Try it, it's almost fun!

The Poison Quiz Book is also designed to be re-used several times to allow, dare we use the word, memorization. A hollow bullet is provided for any scheme of keeping track of questions answered correctly or incorrectly.

We welcome your comments, suggestions, and criticism. Great effort has been made to verify these questions and answers. Some answers may not be the answer you would prefer. Most often this is attributable to variance between original sources. Please make us aware of any errors you find. We hope to make continuous improvements and would greatly appreciate any input with regard to format, organization, content, presentation, or about specific questions. We also are interested in recruiting new contributing authors and publishing new textbooks. We look forward to hearing from you!

Study hard and good luck!

J.H.T. III

ACKNOWLEDGMENTS

The author would like to thank his many colleagues in toxicology, who over the years have contributed questions to be considered for this volume.

PREFACE

Ever since the earliest human first made the connection between the cause and effect relationship of poisons on living things, the subject of poisons has always remained surrounded by both fascination and mystery. Down through the centuries, the subject of poisons has been intermingled with literature, the arts, history, and medicine.

This work is an attempt to present interesting toxicological facts that are intended to challenge, as well as ultimately teach, the reader about the fascinating role poisons have played throughout our history.

These questions were gathered by the author from his perusal of hundreds of international reference works over the last 30 years, in the areas of history, the arts, and toxicology. It is hoped that the contents will prove enjoyable not only to health care professionals, but also to historians, and trivia buffs worldwide.

John Harris Trestrail III, *RPh, FAACT, DABAT*

TABLE OF CONTENTS

ANIMALS

○ Scientists call this snake *Agkistrodon piscivoris leukostoma*. By what more common name is it known?

"Cotton Mouth" or *"Water Moccasin."*

○ What is the common name of the snake native to North America, which toxicologically is most related to the *Cobra* and the *Krait*?

The *"Coral Snake."*

○ Because of their diet, sea otters often have purple colored skeletons. What toxic animal ingredient in their diet causes this color change?

Sea urchins.

○ When the French were testing nuclear weapons in the Sahara, what type of venomous animal was able to withstand the most radiation?

Scorpions.

○ So prevalent are these poisonous living things, that it is estimated there are 2.2 million of them per acre of grassy field. In Britain, it has been estimated they annually consume a mass of prey equivalent to the weight of the human population of the British Isles. What do we commonly call these numerous venomous creatures?

Spiders.

○ We have often heard stories about *"Spanish Fly,"* but what is the biological source of this material?

It is the ground up dried bodies of the "Blister Beetle," *Cantharis vesicatoria.*

○ *"Widow"* is to *Latrodectus*, as what is to *Loxosceles*?

"Recluse." They are part of the common names of toxic spiders.

○ I gained entry into the United States about 1920, near the port of Mobile, Alabama. Scientifically I belong to the genus *Solenopsis*. I have probably the most vicious bite and sting of any other member of my Family. By what common name am I known?

"Fire Ant."

◯   **Do the snakes curled around the staff of *Aesculapius*, the god of medicine, represent venomous or nonvenomous serpents?**

Nonvenomous, the *"Aesculapian Snake."*

◯   **What is the only known natural enemy of the venomous *"Fire Ant"*?**

Man.

◯   ***"Clownfish"* are able to safely live among the venomous stinging tentacles of what marine creatures?**

Sea Anemones.

◯   **Victims who have been stung by the *"Yellow Jacket"* experience the power of a drop of venom. But, is this insect actually a bee or a wasp?**

Wasp.

◯   **In Java there is a Colubrid, or back-fanged, snake known as the *"Fordonia,"* the venom of which is very specialized as to victim. What is so special about this venom?**

It kills the snake's main food source of crabs, yet is harmless to fish and frogs.

◯   **What is the more common name of the southern form of the "Timber Rattlesnake" (*Crotalus horridus*)?**

"Canebrake Rattlesnake."

◯   **The range of the rattlesnake *Crotalus viridis abyssus* is restricted to what popular American tourist attraction?**

The Grand Canyon.

◯   **What is interesting about the venomous fangs of the "Lyre Snakes" (*Trimorphodon bisculatus* subspecies), of the United States?**

They are in the back of the mouth.

◯   **What is unusual about the "Velvet Ant" (*Dasymutilla* species)?**

It is really a wasp.

◯   **Ciguatera gets its name from *"cigua,"* a poisonous creature of the Spanish Antilles. What type of marine creature is it?**

A poisonous Turban Shell.

◯   **What kind of venomous animal is a *"Bearded Gouhl"*?**

A fish, *Inimicus didactylus.*

○   **What is the general medical term used to describe adverse effects caused by butterflies and moths?**

Lepidopterism.

○   **The Italian folk dance known as the *"Tarantella"* was supposedly a cure for the bite of what venomous creature?**

The spider known as the *"tarantula,"* which, by the way, is NOT the same as the banana spider many wrongfully apply the name to today.

○   **Native to Eastern Europe and Asia, they are also found in aquariums as pets. They are species of the genus *Bombina*, which produce the toxins *"bombesin"* and *"bombinine."* What are they more commonly called in English?**

Fire Toads.

○   **Why is a *"Black Widow"* called by that name?**

Because after mating she devours her mate.

○   **The name of what marine related disease comes from the Spanish word for a poisonous marine snail?**

Ciguatera, from the word *"cigua."*

○   **The *Euryterides* was a large scorpion-like creature with a poisonous sting that lived during the Silurian period 440 million years ago. What makes this creature morphologically special?**

At six feet in length, it was the largest invertebrate that ever lived.

○   **Some of the marine fish known as *rays* are venomous, and even newly born ones have a barbed tail which is poisonous. What protects the mother ray from being envenomated by the babies during the birthing process?**

The young are born with their barb flexible in a protective sheath, which is shed after birth.

○   **All of the centipedes are poisonous, but they possess an unusual means of administering their venom. What is it?**

They do not bite, but utilize specialized claws on their front feet.

○   **The manufacturer of *"Black Widow"* spider antivenin uses the venom collected from 28,000 spiders to prepare a bulk batch of this relatively rarely used antidote. This batch will produce enough antivenin to meet the needs of the entire USA, for how many years: 5, 10, or 20?**

5 years.

❍   **The eighth sign of the zodiac, covering the period of October 24th through November 22nd, is based on what toxic animal?**

Scorpio, based on the scorpion.

❍   **What objects have the following names in common: the *Venom*, the *Hornet*, the *Scorpion*, the *Black Widow*, and the *King Cobra*?**

They are all brand names of fixed-wing aircraft.

❍   **This deadly neurotoxin, which causes blockage of nerve impulses and respiratory paralysis, gets its name from the genus of the *Alaskan butter clam*. What is its name?**

Saxitoxin, from *Saxidomus giganteus*.

❍   **How many legs will one find on a scorpion?**

8 legs.

❍   **Most people know that jellyfish can be toxic. But which one is considered to be the most toxic of all?**

"Sea Wasp," *Chironex fleckeri.*

❍   **What popular Italian folk dance was meant to protect the dancers against the bite of dangerous spiders?**

The *"Tarantella."*

❍   **What is unusual about the *"Royal Mayan"* bee?**

It doesn't sting, it bites.

❍   **This marine toxin found in the *Fugu* of Japan is the most toxic non-protein substance found in nature. What is this toxin called?**

Tetrodotoxin.

❍   ***Bufo marinus* is an animal that is capable of releasing a poison when disturbed. What kind of animal is *Bufo marinus*?**

Marine Toad.

❍   **What animal was introduced into *Martinique* to help control the snake population?**

The mongoose.

○   The name of the Cane Toad on display at the Museum of Queensland, Brisbane, Australia, sounds the same as the name of a popular poison prevention character. What is the name?

"Yuck."

○   They are found in phylum Coelenterata, class Anthoza, with over 1,000 species, which include the genera: *Actinia, Physobrachia, Rhodactis, and Sagartia.* What are these toxic things more commonly called?

Anemones.

○   Endotoxins found in the dinoflagellates *Ptychodiscus brevis*, cause *"red tides"* in the Gulf of Mexico, with deleterious effects on fish, shore animals and man. As a group, what are these toxins called?

Brevetoxins.

○   By what regal name is the poisonous *"hamadryad"* better known?

"King Cobra."

○   What host animal is used for the production of the antidote *Digibind*®?

The sheep.

○   To identify venomous snakes responsible for bites, the Australians use something called an *"ELISA"* kit. What does the acronym stand for?

Enzyme-Linked Immunosorbent Assay.

○   We have all heard that all rattlesnakes have rattles, but there is a species of rattlesnake that does NOT possess a rattle. What island is the natural home of this peculiar pit viper?

Santa Catalina Island, Mexico, habitat of *Crotalus catalinensis.*

○   An explorer on a trip to South America was badly bitten by a hemipterous animal. What bit him?

A bug. Bugs belong to the Order "Hemiptera"; the Order belongs to the Class "Insecta."

○   Only one species of scorpion native to North America has been associated with fatality. What is the scientific name of this species of scorpion?

Centruroides exilicauda, (formerly known as *C. sculpturatus*).

○   When a rattlesnake makes a noise with his rattles, what is the musical pitch of the sound that is produced?

Between C and C# (128-135 vibrations/second).

○   **Which of the following insects inject the most venom into a wound: wasp, hornet, yellow jacket, or honeybee?**

The hornet.

○   **I am a venomous resident of most houses preferring to live in dark areas which are damp. I have special poison bearing claws. I may have from 15 to 173 pairs of legs depending on what species I belong to. What common name do I go by?**

Centipede.

○   **Which of the following snakes is NOT a pit viper: Copperhead, Cottonmouth, Boa constrictor, or Rattlesnake.**

Boa constrictor.

○   **A mnemonic device for coral snakes in North America states that the color red is bounded by what color, on the snake's body?**

Yellow or White, remembered by *"Red on yellow or white, kill a fellow or might."*

○   **The venom of what North American rattlesnake contains a major neurological component?**

"Mojave Rattlesnake," *Crotalus scutulatus*

○   **What is the only known member of the *Hymenoptera* group which leaves its stinger behind after the act?**

The honeybee, *Apis mellifera*.

○   **Ancrod (Arvin) a defibringenating enzyme used in medicine as an antithrombotic agent, is derived from the venom of what Asian snake?**

The "Malayan Pit Viper," *Agkistrodon rhodostoma*.

○   **Of the approximate 120 species of snakes in the United States, how many of the species are known to be venomous: 21, 31, or 41?**

21 species.

○   **This particular toxin associated with the ingestion of a variety of shore or reef fishes, shows a distinctive feature of reversal of hot/cold sensations. What is this particular toxin called?**

Ciguatoxin.

○   **The *"Kokoi"* frog of Columbia finds what use by the native indigenous peoples?**

To prepare poisoned arrows, *"Arrow-poison Frog."*

❍   **What venomous snake is said to be the *"Horned Viper"* of the *Book of Genesis* in the *Bible*?**

The "False Cerastes," *Pseudocerastes fieldii.*

❍   **In the parlance of the American Old West, what was *"tarantula juice"*?**

The term for whisky, which was taken orally to treat the bite of these spiders.

❍   **Of the 21 species of venomous snakes in the United States, how many are members of the pit-viper sub-family?**

17 out of 21, or 81%.

❍   **An unusual club exists, where qualification for membership is having been bitten by a venomous snake. What is the official name of this select group?**

The *"White Fang Club."*

❍   **Of the 3,000 known species of snakes in the world, approximately what per cent are venomous: 10%, 25%, or 33%?**

10%.

❍   **What kind of venomous snake did the military name a missile after?**

"Sidewinder."

❍   **In the 15th and 16th centuries, the tusk of the Narwal was worth ten times its weight in gold. Of what use was it to the people of that time?**

They believed that when powdered, it served as a poison detector and antidote.

❍   **This creature was considered the protector of animals because it would supposedly purify a poisoned water hole by dipping its horn into the water, rendering fit to drink. Which creature was it?**

The unicorn.

❍   **We all know that members of genus *Physalia*, commonly known as the *"Portuguese Man-o-war"* are toxic, but where did they ever get that common name?**

The similarity of the body and long tentacles to a Portuguese admiral's hat.

❍   **Peter Parker became a comic book super-hero after being bitten by what toxic creature?**

A radioactive spider.

❍   We all know the bite of the rattlesnake may be poisonous, but how much do you know about the snake itself? Answer the following: (a) The sight of the snake is good to a maximum of how many feet, (b) What ambient temperatures are usually the maximum and minimum for the snake to be normally active, (c) What is the function of the snake's *Jacobson's* organs, (d) Is the hearing of the snake: better, the same, or worse, than in the human?

(a) 15 feet, (b) Maximum = 37 degrees Centigrade (or 98 degrees Fahrenheit), Minimum = 5 degrees Centigrade (or 41 degrees Fahrenheit), (c) Located in the roof of the mouth, they analyze odor molecules picked up from the air and deposited by the snake's tongue, (d) Worse. They are deaf to airborne sounds.

❍   Recent reports from Australia indicate that the drug culture has found a new animal source of hallucinogenic compounds. By boiling the creatures in water and drinking the sludge, there is supposed to follow an *LSD*-like experience. What is the common name of this animal?

The "Cain Toad," *Bufo marinus*.

❍   Many countries have snakes. What is the word for snake in the following languages: (a) German, (b) French, (c) Spanish, (d) Italian, and (e) Japanese.

(a) *schlange*, (b) *serpent*, (c) *serpiente*, (d) *serpente*, (e) *hebi*.

❍   Having a fear of snakes, but wishing to take a trip to other lands, you suggest an itinerary to your travel agent that will include only island countries that have no native snakes. Name the only three such countries that have no native snakes.

Iceland, Ireland, and New Zealand.

❍   Man has only been able to domesticate only two insects. One is venomous and the other is not. Name these domesticated insects.

The Honeybee, *Apis mellifera*, and the Silk Worm, *Bombyx mori*.

❍   Quite a stir was caused in the toxinology world in 1992, when it was reported that the first species of poisonous bird had been identified. Answer the following questions about this unique animal: (a) What is the name of this jungle bird, (b) In what country can this bird be found, (c) Where are the toxic compounds located in the bird's body, (d) What is the name of the toxic compound identified, (e) What two brilliant colors identify this bird, (f) What other known animal contains the same toxins?

(a) "Hooded Pitohui" (pronounced *"PIT-o-hooey"*), (b) Papua New Guinea, (c) feathers, skin, and muscle, (d) Homobatrachotoxin, (e) Orange and black, (f) the "arrow-poison frogs."

❍   If you were working in a poison center in certain countries, you might take a call involving a venomous snake that has the most northern or southern range of any other species of snake in the world. For each snake, name the country: (a) **"European Viper,"** *Vipera burus* - the most northern species, (b) **"Snout-headed Lance Head,"** *Bothrops ammodytoides* - the most southern species.

(a) Norway, (b) Argentina.

○   Multitudes of animals have group names to describe them, such as *"pride"* of lions. What group names are used to describe the following groups known to contain some toxic members: **(a) ants, (b) bees, (c) caterpillars, (d) insects, (e) snakes, and (f) toads.**

(a) *Colony*, (b) *Grist, hive,* or *swarm*, (c) *Army*, (d) *Swarm*, (e) *Bed*, (f) *Knot*.

○   Tell whether the following are physical characteristics of pit-vipers or nonpoisonous snakes in North America: (a) elliptical pupils, (b) subcaudal plates in double rows, and (c) lanceolate shaped heads.

(a) Pit-vipers, (b) Non-poisonous, (c) Pit-vipers.

○   There are only two known venomous lizards. What are the scientific, or common names for each of these lizards?

"Gila Monster," *Heloderma suspectum*, and "Mexican Beaded Lizard," *Heloderma horridum.*

○   Many foreign laboratories produce antivenins. Give the country where each of the following antivenin producers are located: **(a) *Pasteur Institute*, (b) *Haffkine Institute*, (c) *Rizal Institute*, (d) *SAMIR*, (e) *Commonwealth Serum Laboratories*.**

(a) France, (b) India, (c) Republic of the Philippines, (d) South Africa, (e) Australia.

○   Give the continent which is the natural home to the following venomous snakes: (a) *Gaboon Viper*, (b) *Taipan*, (c) *Bushmaster*, (d) *Vipera burus, and (e)* Boomslang.

(a) Africa, (b) Australia, (c) South America, (d) Europe, (e) Africa

○   Indicate whether each of the following statements is *TRUE* or *FALSE*: (a) There are no known venous turtles, (b) There are no known poisonous frogs, (c) Almost all spider are venomous, (d) There are no known venomous mammals, (e) There are no known venomous birds?

(a) True, (b) False, (c) True, (d) False, (e) False.

○   Of all species of rattlesnakes, only two popular names do NOT use the term *"rattlesnake"* in the name. What are the common names for these two snakes?

"Sidewinder," and *"Massasauga."*

○   Name the only four known venomous mammals that are still found in nature.

Platypus, Echidna, Shrew, and Solendon.

❍   **There is only one continent in the world that has no venomous snakes, in fact it has no snakes at all. What is it?**

Antarctica.

❍   **The ancient Egyptians even believed that their gods were susceptible to poisons. Identify each of the following: (a) The *"sun god,"* who nearly died from a snakebite, and (b) The son of *Isis*, who died from the sting of a scorpion.**

(a) *Ra*, (b) *Horus*

❍   **The most venomous of all the snails, are included in what group?**

The "Cone" shells, Family *Conidae*.

❍   **What butterfly concentrates toxic compounds from the *Milkweed* plant, which makes eating them a distasteful experience for predators?**

The "Monarch," *Danaus plexippus*.

❍   **What butterfly, in an example of *Batesian* mimicry, looking like an inedible butterfly, in order to protect itself from potential predators?**

The "Viceroy," *Limentis archippus*.

❍   **This salamander, according to mythology was believed to be immune from heat and fire, and their skin was believed to be made of asbestos. They can spray a toxic secretion from glands along the middle of their backs. What is the more popular name of these animals?**

"Fire Salamanders."

❍   **Which venomous fish has the largest venom gland of any fish, and is such a hazard that an antivenin has been prepared to treat its stings?**

The "Stonefish," *Synanceja horrida*, of Australia.

❍   **For which of the U.S. "Coral" snakes, is the currently available antivenin NOT effective?**

Arizona, or Sonoran Coral Snake (*Micrurus euryxanthus*).

❍   **The most dangerous pit viper in Asia, is found in the *Ryukyu Ilands*, and is marked with a wavy band of dark green blotches. What is the common or scientific name of this snake?**

The "Habu," *Trimeresurus flavoviridis*.

○   The *Cyanea capillata*, is considered the giant among the jellyfish, measuring more than 8 feet across, and with tentacles sometimes 100 feet long. By what more common name is this jellyfish known?

"Lion's Mane Jellyfish."

○   What is the smallest Crotalid snake in the United States?

"Pygmy Rattlesnake," *Crotalus miliarius.*

○   According to many medical experts, what is the most effective thing to carry in your pocket, for use in case of rattlesnake bite?

A set of car keys, to drive the patient to the nearest medical facility, since almost all bites occur within 30 minutes of medical help.

○   A caller to the poison center says he has been stung by the jellyfish known as the *"Portuguese man-o-war."* What is technically incorrect about this statement?

It is not a single animal jellyfish, but a specialized hydrozoan colony of multiple animal polyps.

○   The spider *Atrax robustus*, found in the Southern Pacific region, has a common name associated with what large city?

Sydney, Australia. The *"Sydney Funnel Web Spider."*

○   In South America, the close cousin of our "Brown Recluse" spider, *Loxosceles laeta*, is referred to as *"Arana de detras de los cuadros."* What does this literally mean in Spanish, that describes a common habitat for this creature?

"Spider behind the pictures."

○   A painting by Fra Angelico, in the museum of San Marco located in the city of Florence, shows Christ carrying the Cross, surrounded by three Roman soldiers wearing tunics ornamented with what venomous animals?

Scorpions.

○   In South Africa, this venomous snake is commonly known as the *"Shadow of Death."* By what common or scientific name is this snake known to herpetologists?

The "Black Mamba," *Dendroaspis polylepis.*

○   The *"Black Widow"* spider belong to genus *Latrodectus*. What is the derivation of this Latin name?

It means *"secret biter."*

○   This spider Genus *Phidipus*, contains over 300 species, and the members have excellent eyesight, a body covered with colored hairs, and fluorescent green mouth parts. What are the members of this spider Genus commonly called?

"Jumping Spiders."

○   In the Bible, it is believed that the passage *"These ye shall eat of all that are in the waters; all that have fins and scales ye eat; and whatsoever hath not fins and scales ye may not eat; it is unclean unto you.,"* is thought to warn about the toxic effects of tetrodotoxin. In what book of the *Bible* does this warning occur?

"Deuteronomy," 14:9-10.

○   Venomous stinging cells are found on many marine animals. What is the technical name of this venomous weapon?

"nematocyst."

○   They come in varieties known as: *White, Black, Tam-o-shanter*, and *Long-spined*. What is this group of venomous animals more commonly called?

Sea urchins.

○   By the laws of aerodynamics as demonstrated by wind tunnel tests, this creature is supposed to be unable to fly. Yet, what flying venomous insects prove them all wrong?

Bumblebees.

○   The "Pajaroello" (*Ornithodorus coriaceus*), produces a painful bite due to its toxic saliva. What kind of animal is it?

A Tick.

○   Butterflies of genus *Heloconius*, are known as poisonous pollen feeders, which increases their chances of survival from natural predators. What type of plant compound are they able to incorporate which gives them this protection?

Cyanide compounds.

○   The only living thing visible from space, is a collection of marine organisms, many of which can be toxic. What is this very large structure called?

The *"Great Barrier Reef,"* of Australia.

○   According to diver Jean-Michel Cousteau, what toxic marine animal does their famous divers worry most about when they exploring under water?

Sea urchins.

O   **What kind of snake with more than 50 species, makes them the most common reptile?**

Sea Snakes.

O   **It is considered one of the most toxic marine animals known, and its Genus name comes from a combination of the Greek and Latin for *"murdering hand."* Found in the waters of Australia, what is it more commonly called?**

"The Box Jellyfish," *Chironex fleckeri.*

O   **Species of animals show differences in their tolerance to poisonous substances. What animal is immune to ingested botulinus toxin, but can die after eating just a few green cockle-burrs?**

The swine.

O   **For years the Japanese people used the dried marine annelid worm *Lumbriconereis heteropoda*, as a source of the toxin *Nereistoxin*, to combat what domestic pests?**

Flies.

O   **The Mediterranean mollusc, *Tonna galea*, when irritated, is able to spit/secrete solutions containing approximately 3% of what corrosive material?**

Sulfuric acid.

O   **In 1995, it was reported that a threat of possible extinction existed in Australia, to the *"Cairn's Birdwing"* butterfly from their mistaken utilization of a toxic object. What was the cause of the problem?**

They were laying their eggs on a poisonous vine which, had been imported from Brazil.

O   **What toxic animal has the slowest metabolism of any known invertebrate?**

The scorpion.

O   **What toxic animal has the highest metabolism of any known vertebrate?**

The shrew.

O   **Some of the members of this toxic group of animals include: *"Saddle Back," "Gypsy," "Puss,"* and *"Io."* What is this group commonly called?**

Caterpillars.

O   **Looking at the menu in a Caribbean restaurant, which one of the following fish dishes have been associated with problems with ciguatoxin: Pufferfish, Tuna, Grouper, or Trout?**

Grouper, *Cephalopholis* spp.

○   **In 1991, toxic *Domoic acid* was found in anchovies along the California coast. What animals were becoming victims to this marine toxin?**

Pelicans.

○   **What venomous snake is considered to occupy more land area than any other poisonous snake?**

Vipera berus, "European Viper."

○   **What fish is considered Europe's most venomous?**

The "Weeverfish," *Echiichtys spp.*

○   **There is a type of fly referred to as a *"Bluebottle,"* but what kind of toxic marine organism also bears this common name?**

A jellyfish, *Physalia* spp.

○   **Biologically Cone shells belong to the superfamily *"Toxoglosia,"* what does this name literally mean?**

"poison tongue."

○   **What marine creatures love to feed on jellyfish so much that they continue to feed even after their faces become swollen from the effects of the jellyfish's tentacles?**

Sea Turtles.

○   **The only species of snake that builds a nest, is an extremely venomous one. What snake is it?**

The "King Cobra," *Ophiophagus hannah.*

○   **Rattlesnakes are NOT the only ones that can produce a warning sound. What snake of the world, produces a sound by rasping its body together to produce such a warning?**

The "Saw-scaled Viper," *Echis carniatus.*

○   **The battle began in May, 1996. The Federal government used poisoned margarine on bread, and the activists used tuna and charcoal filter sandwiches. What specific animals were the targets of all their activities?**

"Great Black-backed" and *"Herring"* gulls, Cape Cod, Massachusetts.

○   **Which venomous snake has the largest geographic distribution world wide?**

Vipera berus, "European Viper."

○ **Which Western hemisphere country has more species of venomous snakes than any other country in the Americas?**

Mexico.

○ **Which snake probably kills more people in Africa than any other?**

"Puff Adder," *Bitis arietans.*

○ **Which snake in Cental America causes the most number of bites, many of which are fatal?**

"Barba Amarilla," *Bothrops asper.*

○ **Haiti, the Dominican Republic, and Cuba, are home to the only two species of what venomous mammal?**

"Solendon."

○ **What animal before eating a toad, chews the secretions from the prey's skin into a froth, which is then licked onto its spines, which increases their defensive posture?**

Hedgehogs.

○ **The earliest report of envenomation by this creature was in 866 AD, when the troops of Emperor Ludwig were afflicted in Calabria, Italy. What animal was involved in this incident?**

The "Black Widow" spider, *Latrodectus m. tredecimguttatus.*

○ **A 1996 study from the *Ehime University* in Japan showed that the compound *"TBT,"* found in antifouling paints to prevent barnacles, has also caused the deaths of porpoises, dolphins, and whales in the North Atlantic since the 1980s. What is *"TBT"*?**

Tributyl tin.

○ **In June, 1993, 249 Boa constrictors died from a Cocaine overdose. How were they exposed?**

They were used as *"body packers,"* to smuggle 80 pounds of Cocaine filled condoms into Miami from Bogata, Columbia.

○ **In September 1996, the Australian *RSPCA* awarded the *"Purple Cross Bravery"* medal to *"Fizo,"* a fearless 8-year-old silky terrier. The dog had saved his 9-year-old owner from what toxicological encounter?**

It jumped on, and killed, a 5-foot long *"Brown Snake,"* which was about to strike the young boy.

❍   **In ancient Rome, what animal was considered to be the most venomous, capable of wiping out whole nations at one time?**

The salamander.

❍   **What is the largest spider native to Europe?**

Lycosa trantula, "Wolf Spider."

❍   **What is the only known coelenterate that is lethal to humans?**

Chironex fleckerii, "Box Jellyfish."

❍   **What is the common or scientific name, of the species of snake which is the longest pit viper in the world, as well as the longest venomous snake in the Americas?**

"The Bushmaster," *Lachesis muta.*

❍   **What toxic marine animal's hieroglyphic inscription *"chept"* can be found in several *Fifth Dynasty* Egyptian tombs?**

The "Puffer Fish," *Tetraodon stellatus.*

❍   **The number of species of cantharidin-containing beetles in the world is approximately 15, 150, or 1,500?**

1,500

❍   **The only other creatures on earth, besides man, that make war are also venomous animals. What kind of animals are they?**

Ants.

❍   **What part of the human body is most commonly bitten by insects?**

The foot.

○ Answer this question about the geographic distribution of a type of venomous snake: (a) What is the only genus of "pit vipers," that is found in both the "*Old World*" and the "*New World*," (b) What is the only genus of "pit vipers," that is only found in the "*Old World*"?

(a) *Agkistrodon*, (b)*Trimeresurus*.

○ Not all Black Widow spiders are totally black. Give the color of the following species of *Latrodectus*: (a) *bishopi*, (b) *geometricus*?

(a) *"Red,"* (b) *"Brown."*

○ Rattlesnakes are found native in every state in the United States, except which four states?

Alaska, Delaware, Hawaii, and Maine.

○ Most of the over 30,000 species of spiders are venomous, but the *World Health Organization* lists only four spider genera as responsible for severe human poisoning. List the four genera.

(a) *Atrax,* (b) *Latrodectus*, (c) *Loxosceles*, (d) *Phoneutria*.

○ What marine creature ingests the stinging cells from the coral, and then passes them unharmed to it's skin, to produce a poisonous defense?

The Sea Slug.

○ What is the only American rattlesnake species with prominently raised scales over its eyes, which look like horns?

The Sidewinder, *Crotalus cerastes*.

○ In what country will one find the most number of species of rattlesnakes?

Mexico.

○ What species of rattlesnake has the widest geographical range, from 24° North to 35° South?

The Neotropical Rattlesnake, *Crotalus durrisus*.

○ What is the rarest species of rattlesnake, with only one specimen ever having been found, near Jalisco, Mexico?

The "Autlan Rattlesnake," *Crotalus lannoni*.

○ What U.S. State harbors the largest, as well as the smallest species rattlesnake?

Florida. Eastern Diamondback *Crotalus adamanteus*, and Florida Pygmy Rattlesnake *Sistrurus millearius barbouri*..

○   **March, 1999, the Supreme Court of this U.S. state, declared that a poisonous snake could be considered a weapon, after a man threatened two police officers with his *Rhinoceros Viper*. In what state did this incident occur?**

Montana.

○   **What is unique about the ocular damage and blindness that occurs in swine from the ingestion of Methanol?**

They don't develop the ocular damage, as it only occurs in primates.

○   **This snake has such common names as *"Trapjaw," "Gapper,"* and *"Lowland Moccasin."* What is its more commonly used name?**

"Cottonmouth."

AUTHORS AND BOOKS

○ She was a British author of detective fiction, many of whose 85 books and 148 short stories dealt with murder by poison. Who was she?

Agatha Christie.

○ In 1978, author John Godey wrote a gripping novel about a *"Black Mamba"* snake that terrorized Central Park in New York City. What was the title of this fascinating work?

The Snake.

○ What book in the *Bible* contains the chapter and verse which lead, in 1909, to the rise of snake handling and poison drinking religious cults in the United States?

Mark 16:17 and 18 - *"And these signs shall follow them that believe: In my name shall they cast out devils; they shall speak with new tongues; they shall take up serpents; and if they drink any deadly thing, it shall not hurt them; they shall lay hands on the sick and they shall recover."*

○ Robert Louis Stevenson, is said to have composed the first draft of *Dr. Jekyll and Mr. Hyde*, in just three days, while undergoing treatment for tuberculosis with a certain drug. What was the name of this amazing drug?

Cocaine.

○ What substance is referred to in this quote from Sir Arthur Conan Doyle: *"Sherlock Holmes took his bottle from the corner of the mantelpiece, and his hypodermic syringe from its neat morocco case...It is* [blank] *he said, a seven-percent solution. Would you like to try it?"*

Cocaine, from the *Sign of Four.*

○ What writer of science fiction wrote a story called *"The Purple Pileus,"* which tells the story of a man who wished to commit suicide but turned his life around under the influence of this mysterious mushroom?

H. G. Wells.

○ What famous American writer, comedian, newspaper man, frequenter of the *"Algonquin Round Table,"* and who died from alcoholism, once replied to a friend who said *"what you are drinking is slow poison,"* with – *"so who's in a hurry?"*

Robert Benchley (1889-1945).

○   The French writer Guy de Maupassant (1850-1893), after experimenting with various drugs, became addicted to what volatile substance?

Ether.

○   In Shakespeare's play, Hamlet's father is murdered by poison. How did the killer administer the poison to the victim?

He poured the poison into the ear of the sleeping king.

○   In the 1982 mystery novel *Fever*, by Robin Cook (pseudonym for Dr. Robert William Arthur), Dr. Charles Martel's daughter has leukemia. What does Dr. Martel feel is the source of his daughter's illness?

His daughter, Michelle, was inhaling benzene from the pond behind her playhouse.

○   Elizabeth Barrett Browning was addicted to it and Berlios romanticized its reverie in his *"Symphonie Fantastique."* What was the name of the popular 19th Century plant substance which so influenced these creative people?

Opium.

○   What American writer penned the following lines in "The Cheerful Abstainer": *"I know some poison I could drink; I've often thought I'd taste it; but Mother bought it for the sink, and drinking it would waste it."*?

Edna St. Vincent Milay.

○   What toxic addiction did the Englishman, Thomas De Quincey confess to?

Drug addiction, in *The Confessions of an English Opium Eater*.

○   In Shakespeare's play *"As You Like It,"* what toxic animal is referred to in the following: *"Sweet are the uses of adversity; which, like the* [blank], *ugly and venomous, wears yet a priceless jewel in his head..."*?

Toad.

○   What writer and philosopher wrote *"a little poison now and then: that maketh pleasant dreams. And much poison at last for pleasant death"*?

Frederich Nietzsche.

○   What lyrical poem did Samuel Taylor Coleridge write in his sleep, while under the influence of opium?

"Kubla Khan."

○   When Gertrude Stein's friend and companion, Alice B. Toklas, had her cookbook first published in America, her most famous recipe was omitted. What was the recipe for?

"Hashish Fudge."

○   Niccolo Machiavelli is believed to have created the character in his famous work *The Prince*, around what famous poisoner?

Cesare Borgia.

○   A popular writer for children and adults, wrote some rather tasteless verbiage from a poisoning point of view, an example is *"L is also for Lye. Do you want a nice red lollipop? Go pour all the lye into the toilet. Now tell Mommy you have eaten the lye (that is a fib or a little white lye). Mommy will take you to the doctor in a taxi cab. After the doctor pumps out your stomach, he will give you a nice red lollipop."* Who was the author of *Uncle Shelby's ABZ Book*, who thought this to be humorous writing?

Shel Silverstein.

○   As a third year medical student, I published my first medical article *"Gelsemium as a Poison,"* in the *British Medical Journal*, in 1879. I went on to become famous as a writer of detective fiction. Who was I?

Sir Arthur Conan Doyle.

○   In the first volume of the popular children's books about Babar the elephant, Babar's father dies from eating what toxic substance?

The mushroom "Fly Agaric," *Amanita muscaria*.

○   Which character by Dr. Seuss, is referred to in song as *"a three decker sauerkraut and toadstool sandwich, with arsenic sauce!"*?

The Grinch.

○   What is the only item toxic to the hero Superman?

Kryptonite.

○   In the 1945, Science Fiction novel, *That Hideous Strength*, a radiologist named Francois Alcasan, cuts his brilliant career short by poisoning his wife. What famous Christian author created this work?

C.S. Lewis.

○   The most translated English writing author is William Shakespeare. But, it may surprise one to know that the second most translated English writing author, dealt often with poisons. Who is this author?

Agatha Christie.

❍   **Name the French novelist who lived from 1871-1922, and who, due to his multiple chemical sensitivities, spent most of his final ten years living in an unventilated cork-lined room, to avoid the odors of guest's colognes and perfumes.**

Marcel Proust.

❍   **In the play *"Hamlet,"* the character Laertes attempts to poison Hamlet. What instrument does he use to administer the poison?**

Laertes poisoned the tip of his sword.

❍   **In the short story *"Rapacinni's Daughter,"* the father of Beatrice makes a poison for her and her lover, Giovanni. After that everything they breathed on was doomed to die. What American literary, was the author of this tale?**

Nathaniel Hawthorne.

❍   **In the play *"Macbeth,"* during a truce Macbeth offers liqueur, containing a poisonous plant, to the Danish troops, causing them to fall into a deep sleep, which lead to their slaughter. What plant was used in this chemical warfare?**

Belladonna.

❍   **What Shakespearean character dies from snake-bite?**

Cleopatra.

❍   **In 1844, a physician and friend of what famous Scottish poet, claimed that the poet had died in 1796, from the effects of mercury that had been administered to treat liver disease?**

Robert Burns.

❍   **A famous poem begins with the line *"My heart aches, and a drowsy numbness pains my sense, as though of hemlock I had drunk..."* We know this poem by the title *"Ode To A Nightingale."* Who was the author?**

John Keats.

❍   **What is the title of the book coauthored by toxicologist Lewis Goldfrank, MD, containing such chapter titles as: *"A Question of Poison," "A Peanut and a Mercury Injection,"* and *"Human Warmth and a Drink of Gasoline"*?**

Emergency Doctor.

❍   **What was the name of the *Pulitzer Prize* winning poet who wrote a poem titled *"Mr. Edwards and the Spider,"* which ends with the words *"How long would it seem*** *burning! Let there pass a minute then, ten, ten trillion; but the blaze is infinite, eternal: this is death, to die and know it. This is the Black Widow, death."*

Robert Lowell.

O   **Agatha Christie used many poisons in her detective fiction. But, what was unusual about the medications *Calmo* and *Serenite*, she used in two of her stories?**

They were fictitious substances.

O   **In Shakespeare's play *"Macbeth,"* Act 2, Scene 3, what substance is being described when a character says *"Lecherie, Sir, it provokes, and unprovokes: it provokes the desire, but it takes away the performance."***

"Drink," or ethanol.

O   **What member of the famous *"Algonquin Roundtable"* was commenting on the work of fellow member Dorothy Parker, when he wrote . *"..so potent a distillation of nectar and wormwood, of ambrosia and deadly nightshade, as might suggest to the rest of us, we write far too much."*?**

Alexander Wolcott.

O   **Ethanol in excess can be harmful, but in what popular newspaper cartoon did characters drink *Kickapoo Joy Juice*, brewed in *Big Barnswell's Skonk Works*, the fumes of which have been known to be lethal?**

"L'il Abner," by Al Capp.

O   **What popular novel by Alexander Dumas contains both murder and suicide by strychnine?**

The Count of Monte Cristo.

O   **What American writer is credited for the lines: *"alcohol, hashish, prussic acid, strychnine are weak dilutions; the surest poison is time."***

Ralph Waldo Emerson.

O   **A 1994 play, by the British writer Lisa Evans, titled *"The Shadow of Light,"* is based on the real life of what famous female poisoner?**

Madeleine Smith (1835-1928).

O   **In what Sherlock Holmes story are the toxic effects of a plant called *Radix pedis diaboli* found?**

"The Devil's Foot."

❍ **What popular writer once said** *"give me a decent bottle of poison and I'll construct the perfect crime."*

Agatha Christie.

❍ **What food did Snow White eat that put her to sleep?**

A poisoned apple.

❍ **Sylvia Plath, the famous Boston-born poetess, in a fit of depression, committed suicide in 1963. How did she do it?**

She put her head in an oven and turned on the gas.

❍ **In the comic strips, *"Little Orphan Annie,"* has passed through the years with the help of many protectors. Along with *"Daddy War Bucks,"* and *"Punjab,"* this protector with a venomous name has often saved Annie. Who is he?**

"The Asp."

❍ **What now famous toxicologist of old penned the following:** *"Is not a mystery of nature concealed even in poison?...What has God created that He did not bless with some great gift for the benefit of man? Why then should poison be rejected and despised, if we consider not the poison but its curative virtue?"*

Paracelsus, *Seven Defenses*.

❍ **Who wrote** *"What is food to one man may be fierce poison to others"*?

Lucretius (95-55 B.C.), in *De Rerum Natura*.

❍ **From what Shakespearean play does the following quotation originate:** *."..but let they spiders, that suck up they venom, and heavy-gaited toads lie in their way, doing annoyance to the treacherous feet...yield stinging nettles to mine enemies; and when they from they bosom pluck a flower, guard it, I pray thee, with a lurking adder, whose double tongue may with a mortal touch throw death upon they sovereign's enemies."*?

"Richard the Second" Act 3, Scene 2. Richard speaking.

❍ **In 1869, there was published in New York, a book titled *Micro-Chemistry of Poisons*, by Theo. Wormley. What was the toxicological significance of this book?**

It was the first book published in the United States which dealt totally with the subject of toxicology.

❍ **Alexander Duma's Count of Monte Cristo was addicted to what drug, and used it to drug Maxmillian Morel before reuniting him with Valantine Villefort?**

Hashish.

○   In her 1989, surreal novel *Geek Love*, authoress Katherine Dunn writes about a traveling freak show. Its owners, Al and Lil Binewski, find a novel method of cutting costs in obtaining new performers. What incredible method did they use?

Lil pops pills, injects drugs, and inhales insecticides during ovulation and pregnancy. As a result, her children are born with serious physical deformities.

○   In the 1978 mystery novel *Waxwork*, by Peter Lovesey, the victim Josiah Perceval, is murdered with what poison?

Potassium cyanide.

○   The French writer Guy de Maupassant (1850-1893), after experimenting with various drugs became addicted to what volatile substance?

Ether.

○   In 1966, author Ed McBain wrote a novel titled *Eighty Million Eyes*, in which a poison plays a part. What poison is it?

Strophanthin.

○   A science fiction classic uses poisons and poisoners in many of the interactions between its *"spacey"* characters. What is the title of this work by author Frank Herbert?

Dune.

○   The French author Charles Baudelaire (1821-1867), was one of the first of the *"Decadents."* In his 1860 work *Les Paradis Artificiels*, he described his experiences under what mind-altering substance?

Hashish. He was a member of *"Le Club des Hashicians"* in Paris.

○   What drug was abused by the character Mary Tyrone in Eugene O'Neill's *"Long Day's Journey into Night"*?

Morphine.

○   In 1947, Aldous Huxley published *The Doors of Perception* in which he described his experiences under what hallucinogenic agent?

Mescaline.

○   The only mention in the *Bible*, actually the books collectively called the *"Apochrypha,"* of suicide by a poisonous agent was that of Ptolemeus, who *"…departed to Anthiochus Epiphanes, and seeing that he was in no honorable place, he was so discouraged that he poisoned himself and died."* In what book of the early *Bible* will one find this reference?

II Macabes, Chapter X, verse 13.

○   **In 1702, there was published the first book in English devoted entirely to poisons. The work was titled *The Mechanical Account of Poisons*. Who was the celebrated physician author?**

Richard Mead, M.D. (1673-1754).

○   **In his work *Paradise Lost*, Milton describes a serpent named *"Dipsas,"* the bite of which resulted in symptoms different from our snakes of today. What happened to people bitten by this snake?**

They suffered from intolerable thirst.

○   **What drug of abuse figures in William Burrough's *The Naked Lunch*?**

Heroin.

○   **A humorous mystery drama play was written by Russel Crouse and Howard Lindsay, which had 1,444 performances. What was the name of this popular play which involved, the use of a metallic poison?**

"Arsenic and Old Lace."

○   **In Thomas Hardy's novel *The Return of the Native*, Mrs. Yeobright, the mother of the main character, is mortally bitten by what kind of snake?**

An "adder," *Vipera berus.*

○   **Of what hallucinogenic plant did Carlos Casteneda's Don Juan claim expert knowledge?**

Peyote.

○   **In a 1982 mystery novel by Dick Francis, a poison was given to mares in apples that would cause their foals to be deformed. What was the poisonous element?**

Selenium.

○   **In this literary work a small girl had many strange adventures, and one will find the quote *"She has never forgotten that, if you drink much from a bottle marked `poison', it is almost certain to disagree with you, sooner or later."* What is the title of this ever popular work?**

Alice in Wonderland, by Lewis Carroll.

○   **Patrick Branwell Bronte, the brother and tutor of the famous sister authoresses: Anne, Charlotte, and Emily; was addicted to what crude plant substance?**

Opium.

○   **In a mystery novel titled *Red Harvest*, a town named *Personville* (but pronounced *Poisonville*) is taken over by criminals. What is the name of the famous mystery writer of this novel?**

Dashiell Hammett.

○   **Who was the Austrian playwright, author, and biographer (best known for his psychological portraits of literary and historical characters), who died with his wife Lotte, in a suicide pact, by taking the drug Veronal® (Barbital)?**

Stefan Zweig (1881-1942).

○   **In 1984, an argument was put forth that the death in 1784, of what famous English writer, was hastened by an accidental overdose of digitalis administered by his physician?**

Dr. Samuel Johnson.

○   **Imogen is poisoned by her wicked stepmother, which caused a comatose state, in which work by Shakespeare?**

"Cymbaline."

○   **In 1991, Derek Humphrey authored a book which was a suicidal primer for euthanasia. Some of the advice involved poisons. What was the title of this controversial work?**

Final Exit.

○   **In 1991, the book *Poison Pen* appeared which was the unauthorized biography of what sensational biographer of the time?**

Kitty Kelly.

○   **In the 1989 best seller *Clear and Present Danger*, by Tom Clancy, we read of the "suicidal" overdose of Moira Murray. With what drug was the deed carried out?**

Placidyl®, or Ethchlorvynol.

○   **What famous Russian writer's death in 1936, was hastened by the murderous administration of camphor, digitalis, and strychnine?**

Maxim Gorky (1868-1936).

○   **In 1992, the New York publisher Ballantine Books had to recall all November 1991 copies of its *"Great Cakes"* recipe collection, by Carol Walter, because on page 499, it had suggested decorating the desserts with what toxic flower?**

"Lilly-of-the-Valley."

○   **I won a Pulitzer Prize in 1966 for the book *Live or Die*. I was a friend of the tragic suicidal author Sylvia Plath, and in a similar way I ended my life in 1974, by gassing myself in a garage. Who was I?**

Anne Sexton.

○   **What English writer composed an essay on the 19th Century poisoner Thomas Wainewright, titled *Pen, Pencil and Poison*?**

Oscar Wilde.

○   **In 1970, Peter Lovesey, wrote a mystery novel titled *Wobble to Death*. Situated at a race track, the front-runner in the races was killed with what poisonous substance?**

Strychnine.

○   **Colleen McCullough, in her novel *The First Man in Rome*, writes about the death of a female character named *Nicopilis*, from a toxic agent called *"The Destroyer."* What was the source of this fatality?**

Mushrooms.

○   **Here are three clues to the identity of a famous drug addicted author. FIRST CLUE: I was born on January 19, 1809, and was a literary figure of renown, but my life was adversely affected by my addiction to ethanol and opium. SECOND CLUE: I was expelled from the academy at West Point in 1831, because of my conduct. THIRD CLUE: I am described by many as the *"father"* of the detective story. Who was I?**

Edgar Allan Poe.

○   **Shakespeare wrote often about the use of poisons in his plays. Give the name of the play from which each of the following quotations are taken: (a) *"Let me have a dram of poison, such soon-speeding gear as will disperse itself through all the veins. That the life-weary taker may fall dead, and that the trunk may be discharg'd of breath as violently as hasty powder fir'd doth hurry from the fatal cannon's womb.,"* (b) *"Poison'd -- ill fare! Dead, forsook, cast off; and none of you will bid the winter come to thrust his icy fingers in my maw, not let my kingdom's rivers take their course through my burn'd bosom, nor entreat the north to make his bleak winds kiss my parched lips and comfort me with cold.,"* (c) *"Upon my secure hour they uncle stole, with juice of cursed hebenon in a vial, and in the porches of mine ears did pour this leperous distilment...,"* (d) *"In poison there is physic."***

(a) *Romeo and Juliet*, V.i.59, (b) *King John*, V.vii.34, (c) *Hamlet*, I.v.61, (d) *King Henry IV*, Part II I.i.137.

○ **There are many references to poison in literature. Name the author of the following literary lines: (a) *"The strongest poison ever known, came from Caesar's Laurel crown.,"* (b) *"The surest poison is time.,"* (c) *"In every man's heart there springs in the end. This poison that he cannot trust a friend."***

(a) William Blake (1757-1827) in *Augeries of Innocence*, (b) Ralph Waldo Emerson (1803-1882), (c) Aeschylus (525-456 B.C.).

○ **Mystery writers often make references to poisons in their works. Identify the author or the work from which each of the following quotations originate: (a) *"A man who can listen at doors -- is worse than a poisoner.,"* (b) *"Confidence is a good thing...but conceit is a mortal poison.,"* (c) *"Love is like a mushroom. No roots and deadly poison.,"* (d) *"The best way to kill a food taster is by poisoning his master's dish."***

(a) *Bastard Verdict,* by Winifred Duke, (b) *Burial Service*, by Paul McGuire, (c) *No Match for Murder*, by Jean Francis Webb, (d) *The Alamak Ambush*, by Anthony Price.

○ **And now to see how well you know Shakespearian characters and how they met their deaths. Indicate whether each of the following characters met they deaths by poison or not: (a) Othello, (b) Hamlet, (c) Romeo, (d) Richard III, (e) MacBeth.**

(a) No, (b) Yes, (c) Yes, (d) No, (e) No.

○ **In many of the adventures of Sherlock Holmes written by Sir Arthur Conan Doyle, poisons figured into the plot. Identify the poison in each of the following adventures: (a) *The Adventure of the Retired Colourman*, (b) *The Adventures of the Sussex Vampire*, (c) *The Adventure of the Speckled Band*, (d) *The Greek Interpreter*, (e) *A Study in Scarlet*.**

(a) Coal gas, (b) Curare, (c) Swamp Adder, (d) Carbon monoxide, (e) Curare.

○ **Tell what poison was used in the following works of fiction in an attempt to do harm: (a) *The Name of the Rose*, by Umberto Eco, (b) *Final Curtain*, by Ngaio Marsh, (c) *Bitter Almond*, by Dorothy Sayers, (d) *Madame Bovary*, by Gustave Flaubert.**

(a) Arsenic, (b) Thallium acetate, (c) Cyanide, (d) Arsenic.

○ **We all know the safety importance of clean food processing, but in 1906, a significant novel was published exposing the meat-packing industry, which prompted the Federal government to pass pure-food legislation. The author changed the public's mind, by turning the public's stomach. (a) Name the author of this sensational work, and (b) Name the title of his book.**

(a) Upton Sinclair, (b) *The Jungle.*

○ **Identify the author of each of the following quotes about poison: (a) *"One sickly sheep infects the flock. And poisons all the rest.,"* (b) *"Our Adonais has drunk*** *poison -- oh!. What deaf and viperous murderer could crown Life's early ways with such a draught of woe?,"* **(c)** *"There is such a thing as legitimate warfare: war has its laws, there are things which may be fairly done, and things which may not be done...He has attempted (as I may call it) to poison the wells.,"* **(d)** *"Let him drink port, the English statesman cried -- He drank poison and his spirit died."*

(a) Isaac Watts (1674-1748), *Against Idleness and Mischief,* (b) Percy Bysshe Shelley (1792-1822), *Adonais,* (c) John Henry, Cardinal Newman (1801-1890), *Apologia suo Vita Sua,* 1864, (d) John Hume, (1722-1808), *Life of Scold.*

❍   **Identify the author of each of the following quotes about poison: (a)** *"And most of all would I flee from the cruel madness of love — The honey of poison-flowers and all the measureless ill.,"* **(b)** *"He crams with can of poisoned meat. The subjects of the King. And when they die by thousands, why, he laughs like anything.,"* **(c)** *"Hope of high talk with the departed dead. I called on poisonous names with which our youth is fed."*

(a) Alfred Lord Tennyson, *Maud,* (b) G. K. Chesterton, *"The Secret People,"* (c) Percy Bysshe Shelley (1792-1822), *"Hymn to Intellectual Beauty."*

❍   **Some authors have penned stories with the name of a poisonous plant in the title. Given the author, provide the title of the story which contains such a plant. (a) Ellis Peters, (b) Jude Deveraux, (c) Agatha Christie, and (d) Eli Sagan.**

(a) *Monkshood,* (b) *Mountain Laurel,* (c) *Yellow Iris,* (d) *The Honey and the Hemlock.*

❍   **For each of the following toxic sounding Marvel Comic characters, state whether they are a hero or a villain: (a)** *"Tarantula,"* **(b)** *"Asp,"* **(c)** *"Black Widow,"* **(d)** *"Cobra,"* **and (e)** *"Scorpion."*

(a) Villain, (b) Villain, (c) Heroine (ex-villain), (d) Villain, (e) Villain.

❍   **In** *Act IV, Scene 1,* **of Shakespeare's** *"The Tragedy of Macbeth,"* **three witches** *"round about the cauldron go"* **preparing a poisonous concoction. What five animals or plants did they mention as ingredients for their magical mixture, that today we know have some toxicological basis for their use?**

"toad...," "eye of newt," "adder's fork," "root of hemlock," and "slips of yew."

❍   **For each of the following fictional characters, state what poisonous agent was used to do them harm. (a) Hamlet's father, (b) James Bond in** *From Russia With Love,* **(c)** *Snow White,* **(d) Clint Eastwood in the movie** *"The Beguiled,"* **(e) Sherlock Holmes in** *"The Speckled Band."*

(a) Henbane, (b) Tetrodotoxin, (c) Poisoned apple, (d) Mushrooms, (e) Swamp Adder.

❍   **In 1962, an author published a popular and now famous work which detailed the effects of toxic chemicals, like** *DDT,* **in the world's environment and food chain.**

Answer the following: (a) What was the title of this prophetic book, and (b) Who was the author?

(a) *Silent Spring*, (b) Rachel Carson.

○   **Agatha Christie was a prolific writer of detective fiction. In each of the following stories written by her, identify which poison was utilized: (a) *The Body in the Library*, (b) *And Then There Were None*, (c) *The House of Lurking Death*, (d) *The Pale Horse*, (e) *The Cretan Bull*.**

(a) Digitalis, (b) Cyanide, (c) Ricin, (d) Thallium, (e) Atropine.

○   **In 1958, the author Jean Plaidy, wrote a book titled *A Triptych of Poisoners*, in which are detailed the lives of three real and infamous homicidal poisoners. What three poisoners are discussed?**

Cesare Borgia, La Marquise De Brinvilliers, and Dr. Edward Pritchard.

○   **What author wrote a poem titled *"In A Dispensary,"* alluding to experiences gained in a Red Cross Hospital dispensary, which includes the line *"And high on the wall, beneath lock and key, the powers of the Quick and the Dead! Little low bottles of blue and green, each with a legend red..."*?**

Agatha Christie.

○   **When Ulysses set out to rescue his followers, Hermes recommends he take an herb called "moli," saying *"Take then the antidote the Gods provide. The plant I give through all the direful power, shall guard thee and avert the evil hour."* Who was the author of this epic tale?**

Homer.

○   **What Greek playwright, a contemporary of Socrates, alluded to the *Athenian State Poison* in his play *"The Frogs"*?**

Aristophanes.

○   **What character created by famous mathematician and writer Charles Dodgson, is thought to show the mind altering effects of occupational Mercury exposure?**

The *"Mad Hatter,"* in *Alice in Wonderland*, created by Lewis Carroll.

○   **What popular English poet of the late 1800s wrote the following: *"It is unjust that when we have done all that a serpent should, you gather our poisons, one by one, and break them down to your good"*?**

Rudyard Kipling.

❍   **In this original play, first performed in 1904, to save her beloved friend a character with the last name of Bell, swallows poison, and is revived when her friend says *"Do you believe in fairies? If you believe, clap your hands!."* In what play by British playwright James Matthew Barrie, did this scene occur?**

"Peter Pan."

❍   **In a work by Harry Leon Wilson, a character states *"She'd fight a rattlesnake and give it the first two bites.* What was the title of this work?**

Ruggles of Red Gap.

❍   **The *Book of Exodus* 7:19-21, in the *Bible*, is thought to be the earliest record of the toxic effects of what marine condition?**

"red tide"

❍   **In the Greek poem *"Cassandra,"* written about 250 B.C., there is a prediction of the death of Ulysses, from a spear tipped with what toxic agent?**

"the sting of a venomous fish," possibly a stingray.

❍   **How about the association of a literary personage with a toxic critter — this British literary figure who lived from 1688-1744, was referred to as the *"Wicked Wasp of Twickenham,"* because of his spiteful and venomous attacks on his contemporaries. The author of the *"Rape of the Lock,"* who was he?**

Alexander Pope.

❍   **Toxicologists know that picking peppers can produce a skin reaction known as *"Hunan Hand."* But what children's nursery rhyme character was able to pick peppers supposedly without bad results?**

Peter Piper, who picked a peck of pickled peppers.

❍   **In this popular children's book, the reader will find a poem telling the story of a young girl named *Goldie Pinklesweet*, who suffers the consequences of eating her grandmother's powerful laxatives. What is the title of this popular book?**

Charlie and the Great Glass Elevator.

❍   **What famous author who's wife died in 1862 from an overdose of laudanum, was so moved by her death that he buried an unpublished manuscript of his writings along with his wife in the casket?**

Dante Gabriel Rossetti.

❍   **Name the first American journal dedicated to the subject of toxicology.**

Toxicology and Applied Pharmacology.

○ *"Lucretia Borgia,"* a play about the believed infamous Italian poisoner, was written by what famous French author?

Victor Hugo.

○ In 1674, this French dramatist, known for the effective simplicity of his poetic style and his psychological portrayals of the passions of his characters, produced a play titled *"Mithridate,"* which told of the tragedy of the poison-antidote creating King Mithridates. What was the name of this dramatist?

Jean Racine (1639-1699).

○ In which novel by author Robin Cook is a new antidepressant, called *"Ultra,"* created from the mold that poisoned the victims of the *Salem Witch Trials*?

Acceptable Risk.

○ In Rudyard Kipling's *The Jungle Book*, the wolves who reared Mowgli called themselves the *"Free People"* Who did they call the *"Poison People"*?

The cobras.

○ In JRR Tolkien's masterpiece, *The Lord of the Rings*, Aragorn saves Faramir, who had been struck by poisoned dart, using the plant *"Kingsfoil."* In which book of the trilogy does this event occur?

The Return of the King.

○ In JRR Tolkien's *The Lord of the Rings*, what is the name of the giant spider, that poisons Frodo on his way into Mordor?

"Shelob."

○ In 1983, what famous writer and journalist, suffering from leukemia, committed suicide with an overdose of barbiturates?

Arthur Koestler.

○ What Shakesperean character makes the following comment: *"Let us sit upon the ground, and tell sad stories of the death of kings: — How some have been deposed, some slain in war; some poisoned by their wives, some sleeping killed; all murdered."*?

Richard II.

○ In what book of the *Bible* does one find the following reference to poisoned arrows: *"For the arrows of the Almighty are within me, the poison whereof drinketh up my spirit..."*?

Job 6:6.

❍ **During the 15th Century, no less than 14 editions of the famous work *De Venenis*, were published. Who was the author of this popular toxicological work?**

Peter Abano.

❍ **The book, by Steven King, involves the created addiction to the opiate drug *Novril*, of author Paul Sheldon, by his obsessed fan Annie Wilkes. What is the title of this popular book made into a film?**

Misery.

❍ **In the *Bible's* Old Testament's *"Book of Kings,"* which prophet turned the poisonous gourd *Colocynthis* ("Bitter Apple"), into an edible plant during a famine in Gilgal?**

Elisha.

❍ **In the 1995 novel *The Lost World*, by Michael Crichton, what potent neurotoxin was used in the impact-delivery darts fired from the *Lindstradt* air guns, to subdue the animal prey?**

Venom of the "South Sea" coneshell, *Conus purpurascens.*

❍ **In this 1905 novel by Edith Wharton, the character Lily Bart dies from an overdose of Chloral hydrate. What is the title of this work with its plot of social criticism?**

The House of Mirth.

❍ **In the famous work *The Canterbury Tales*, by Geoffrey Chaucer (1340?-1400), one of the stories concerns the death of the characters from poisoned wine, in an attempt to obtain a huge pile of gold coins. Which tale tells of this toxicological murder?**

"The Pardoner's Tale."

❍ **What 1844 novel by Charles Dickens involves murder by poison?**

The Life and Adventures of Martin Chuzzlewit.

❍ **What famous American poetess wrote the following: *"Had nature any outcast face? Could she a son condemn? Had nature an Iscariot. That mushroom – it is him."*?**

Emily Dickinson.

❍ **What American poet, who lived from 1879-1931, and who's most famous poems are *"General William Booth Enters Into Heaven,"* and *"Congo,"* committed suicide in 1931, by drinking Lysol?**

Vachel (Nicholas) Lindsay.

❍ **Name the author of the following:** *"Peace upon earth! Was said. We sing it, and pay a million priests to bring it; After two thousand years of mass. We've got as far as poison-gas."*

Thomas Hardy (1840-1928), *"Christmas,"* 1924.

❍ **In his most famous work** *"Elegy in a Country Churchyard,"* **the poet describes a toxic yew planted above the** *"mouldering heaps."* **What English poet wrote this famous poem in 1751?**

Thomas Gray.

❍ **In his poem** *"The Upas Tree,"* **a poet described** *Antiaris toxicaria* **of the Orient, a tree supposedly so toxic that birds were poisoned by merely resting on its branches. Who was the famous Russian poet of this poison related piece?**

Alexander Pushkin.

❍ **What English poet in his poem** *"Ode on Melancholy,"* **wrote the following lines:** *"No, no, got not to Lethe, neither twist — Wolf's-bane, tight-rooted, for its poisonous wine"*?

John Keats.

❍ **The 1943 novel** *Airing in a Closed Baby Carriage*, **by Joseph Shearing, is based upon what infamous poisoner of 1889?**

Florence Maybrick.

❍ **The 1929 novel** *The Poisoned Chocolate Case*, **by Anthony Berkeley, is based upon what real 1898 poisoner?**

Roland Molineaux.

❍ **The 1932 novel** *What Really Happened*, **by Marie Belloc Lowndes, is based upon what real 1876 poison case?**

Florence Bravo.

❍ **The** *"Tale of the Hashish Eater,"* **is a story to be found in what great collection of Arabic stories?**

The Thousand and One Nights.

❍ **In 1854, what American poet wrote about hallucinations caused by hashish in his collection of** *Anti-Slavery Poems*?

John Greenleaf Whittier.

❍   **What famous British writer in 1933, referred to himself as the world's** *"cosmic dentist"* **for his use of Nitrous oxide to treat his toothaches?**

George Bernard Shaw.

❍   **In 1913, a book titled** *The Poison Belt: Being an Account of Another Amazing Adventure of Professor Challenger,"* **was written by what great author of detective fiction?**

Sir Arthur Conon Doyle.

❍   **Should** *"Little Miss Muffet,"* **an acknowledged arachnophobe, while sitting on her tuffet, be afraid of a** *Centruroides exilicauda***?**

Yes, the Scorpion belongs to Class Arachnidia.

❍   **In Aldous Huxley's** *Brave New World,* **what was the name of the social drug which had all the advantages of Christianity and alcohol; none of their defects, and allowed people to take a holiday from reality?**

Soma.

❍   **Produced on record by the** *American Foundation for the Blind,* **this novel tells of the 18th century Scottish murder trial from Thomas Ogilvie dying from poison. What is the title of this work?**

The Case of Kitty Ogilvie.

❍   **Published in 1939, this novel by Elispeth Huxley, tells of the story of Supt. Vachell on the trail of a Nazi bund and a deadly arrow poison. What is the title of this work?**

The African Poison Murders.

❍   **In the popular book** *Midnight in the Garden of Good and Evil,* **what poison is being described by Luther, when he says** *"This is one way out...Five hundred times more lethal than Arsenic"***?**

Sodium monofluoroacetate.

❍   **Poisons have long been a part of mystery writing. Name the fictional detective, who is featured in the work having a toxic reference in the title: (a)** *Monkshood,* **(b)** *Poison,* **(c)** *Poison Ivy,* **(d)** *Nightshades,* **(e)** *Strong Poison***?**

(a) Brother Cadfael, (b) Steve Carella, (c) Lemmy Caution, (d) The Nameless Detective, (e) Lord Peter Wimsey.

❍   **Poisons have long been a part of mystery writing. Name the fictional detective, who is featured in the work having a toxic reference in the title: (a)** *Spotted Hemlock,*

(b) *A Poison That Leaves No Trace*, **(c)** *Sing A Song for Cyanide*, **(d)** *Poison in the Pen*, **(e)** *Poisoned Pins*?

Dame Beatriuce Adela LaStrange Bradley, (b) Kinsey Millhone, (c) Mrs. Palmyra Pym, (d) Miss Maud Hepzibah Silver, (e) Claire Malloy.

○ **Give the author or the title of the piece that contains each of the following quotations that mention poison: (a) Th' adorning thee with so much art is but a dangerous skill; tis like the poisoning of a dart too apt before to kill, (b) There be some men are born only to suck out the poison of books, (c) Because all earth, except his native and, to him is one wide prison, and each breath of foreign air he draws seems a slow poison, consuming but not killing, (d) He who teaches a woman letters feeds more poison to a frightful asp, (e) Venenum in auro bibitur (Poison is drunk from cups of gold).**

(a) Abraham Cowley, *The Waiting Maid*, (b) Ben Johnson, *Explorata: De Maglin, Studentium*, (c) Byron, *The Two Foscari*, Act I, Sc. 1, (d) Menander, *Fragments*, No. 702, (e) Seneca, *Thyestes*, 1. 453.

○ **Give the author or the title of the piece that contains each of the following quotations that mention poison: (a) "Poison is poison though it comes in a golden cup," (b) "They love not poison that do poison need," (c) "Inpia sub dulci melle venena latent" (Wicked poisons lurk in sweet honey), (d) "Cum fata volunt, bina venena juvant" (When the Fates will, two poisons work for good), (e) "Still on that breast enamor'd let me lie, still drink delicious poison from thy eye, pant on thy lip, and to they heart be press'd."**

(a) Thomas Adams, *Works*, (1630), (b) Shakespeare, *Richard II*, Act. V, Sc. 1, l. 333, (c) Ovid, *Amores*, Bk. 1, eleg. 8, l. 104, (d) Ausonius, *Epigrams*, No. iii, l. 12, (e) Alexander Pope, *Eloisa to Abelard*, l. 121.

○ **Give the author or the title of the piece that contains each of the following quotations that mention poison: (a)** *An I have not ballads made on you all and sung to filthy tunes, let a cup of sack be my poison,* **(b)** *There is a snake in thy smile, my dear, and bitter poison within thy tear,* **(c)** *So that Lancashire merchants whenever they like, can water the beer of a man in Klondike, or poison the beer of a man in Bombay; and that is the meaning of Empire day,* **(d)** *The honey-bee that wanders all day long... Seeks not alone the rose's glowing breast, The lilly's dainty cup, the violet's lips, But from all rank of noxious weeds he sips The single drop of sweetness closely pressed Within the poison chalice,* **(e)** *I know too well the poison and the sting of things too sweet.*

(a) Shakespeare, *Henry IV*, Act 2, sc. 2, l. 48, (b) Percy Shelley, *The Cenci: Song*, Act 5, sc. 4, (c) G. K. Chesterton, *Songs of Education*, (d) Anne Botta, *The Lesson of the Bee*, (e) Adelaide Ann Procter, *Per Pacem ad Lucem.*

○ **What author who had won the 1976 Noble Prize for literature, spent five months in an intensive care unit, due to the ingestion of Ciguatera fish poison?**

Saul Bellow.

○   In the book *Curious George Gets a Job*, George is sent to the hospital. While there his curiosity gets the better of him, when he opens a bottle, inhales the contents, and is rendered unconscious. What did the bottle contain that knocked him out?

Ether.

○   Shakespeare only mentions one antidote in his plays. It is Oberon's drug, which removes the pansy's effects. In what play is this antidote mentioned?

Midsummer Night's Dream (III.ii. 366-369).

○   A 1997 novel by Frank Freudberg, concerned a man dying of cancer, who poisons hundreds of packages of cigarettes with Cyanide, and plants them in hundreds of stores, offices, and restaurants around the country, in order to take the tobacco industry down with him. What is the title of this disturbing work?

Gasp! A Novel of Revenge.

○   In the book by J.R.R. Tolkien, the character Bilbo Baggin's mother shared the same name as what toxic plant?

Belladonna Took Baggins.

○   In another James Bond adventure, by author Raymond Benson, the hero is up against an evil secret society called *Decada*, who have stockpiled a range of poisons to use to gain power and revenge. What is the title of this 1998 book?

The Facts of Death.

○   A popular read along book and record, by the Jim Henson Muppets, is titled *"Gobo Fraggle and the Poison* [blank]." What word completes the blank?

Cackler.

○   Give the author or the title of the piece that contains each of the following quotations that mention poison: (a) "Venom destroys venom," (b) "The gnat that sings his summer's song Poison gets from Slander's tongue. The poison of the snake and newt Is the sweat of Envy's foot. The poison of the honey-bee. Is the artist's jealousy...The strongest poison ever known Came from Caesar's laurel crown," (c) "The poisons are our principal medicines, which kill the disease, and save life.," (d) "Quod aliis cibus est, aliis fuat acre venenum" (What to some is food, to others may be sharp poison), and (e) "Wan Lo has made an amazing discovery. "I have found," he cries, "That what is one man's poison, is another man's poison."

(a) Langland, *Piers Plowman*, Passus xxi, l. 156, (b) William Blake, *Auguries of Innocence*, l. 45, (c) Emerson, *Conduct of Life: Considerations by the Way*, (d) Lucretius, *De Rerum Natura*, Bk iv, l. 638, and (e) Henry Harrison, *Wan Lo Tanka*.

CONDITIONS:
PHYSICAL AND MENTAL

○ **A deficiency of this enzyme predisposes certain individuals to severe toxic effects from exposure to naphthalene. What is the short abbreviation of this enzyme?**

G-6-PD.

○ **If the iron atom in the center of the heme molecule is oxidized from the ferrous to ferric state, what is produced?**

Methemoglobin.

○ **By what more common name do we know the condition which is characterized by sudden onset of thirst, chills, myalgias, headache and fever; and results from exposure to a suspension of microscopic oxidized metallic particles?**

"Metal Fume Fever."

○ **Intoxication by what element has been implicated in the pathogenesis of "Alzheimer's" disease?**

Aluminum.

○ **If one is suffering from "mahi-mahi" disease, would the cause be animal, vegetable, or mineral?**

Animal. The *"mahi-mahi"* is the dolphin fish (NOT the mammal) of Hawaii, which can cause ciguatoxin poisonings.

○ **In 1775, the Englishman Sir Percival Pott, first described the presence of scrotal cancer in workers of what occupation?**

Chimney sweeps.

○ **This physical illness which clinical ecologists believe is caused by minute levels of toxic chemicals in the air, water, and food. It is known as *MCS*. What does this acronym stand for?**

Multiple Chemical Sensitivity.

❍   The *"gray baby syndrome"* is the most serious form of toxicity to what drug?

Chloramphenicol.

❍   The *"red man's syndrome"* describes the classic presentation of acute toxicity to what anti-infective drug?

Rifampin, or vancomycin.

❍   The mind-altering condition *"synaesthesia"* is often seen with the use of *LSD.* What happens during this condition?

Transformation of sensations (i.e. music to colors or *vice versa*).

❍   When catechols or alkylating phenols react with the body's tyrosinase in melanosomes, they eventually lead to what medical condition?

Vitiligo, or Leukoderma.

❍   What is the name of the syndrome used to describe the experiences of people living in buildings whose indoor air is heavily contaminated with toxic pollutants?

"Sick Building Syndrome."

❍   The *"Chinese Restaurant Syndrome"* is thought to be due to what culinary chemical?

MSG, or Monosodium glutamate.

❍   Workers exposed to vapors of Trichloroethane or Trichloroethylene may suffer a disulfiram-like effect upon exposure to ethanol. What is the common name for this condition?

"Degreaser's flush."

❍   The phenomenon where toxic substances are intentionally administered by caretakers, to children to produce medical conditions, has become known as what?

"Munchausen Syndrome by Proxy."

❍   Prior to 1950, intoxication by what agent plagued workers involved in the manufacturing of fluorescent lamps?

Beryllium.

❍   In 1966, there occurred in England, a condition known as *"Epping Jaundice,"* which involved 84 patients, who had consumed bread which had been made from flour contaminated in transit by what chemical?

Methylenedianiline.

❍   **In a 1976 issue of the *Journal of the American Medical Association*, what term was used to describe a battery burn resulting from carrying a transistor battery in one's pocket?**

"Hot pants Syndrome."

❍   **The condition known as *"beer drinker's cardiomyopathy"* results from the use of what substance as a beer defoaming agent?**

Cobalt.

❍   **A condition known as *"risus sardonicus"* is associated with intoxication by what substance?**

Strychnine.

❍   **The drug piperazine citrate, used to treat *Ascaris* infestations, is liable to produce severe ataxia and vertigo if administered in excessive doses. The resultant syndrome of acute ataxia in toddlers, is more commonly known as what?**

"Worm wobble."

❍   **Discolorations of the skin can be an important clue to industrial exposures to toxic materials. What discoloration of the skin, would be produced by dermal contact with the following chemicals: (a) Chlorine gas, (b) Picric acid, (c) Copper salts, (d) Oxalic acid, (e) *p*-phenylenediamine, (f) Silver nitrate?**

(a) Orange, (b) Yellow, (c) Green, (d) Blue, (e) Brown, (f) Black.

❍   **Give the three *"street"* terms used to describe methods for abusing volatile solvents by the inhalation route, and describe how each is performed.**

(a) *"Sniffing"* - smelling substance from the original container, (b) *"Huffing"* - breathing substance from an impregnated cloth, (c) *"Bagging"* - breathing substance contained inside a plastic bag.

❍   **State whether each of the following is *TRUE* or *FALSE* as it refers to the psychological profile of these intentional poisoner: (a) Usually has been spoiled by his/her parents, (b) Mind is limited, without sympathy and imagination, (c) Openly accepts a moral basis for life, (d) Lacks vanity - feels he/she can be easily detected in the crime, (e) Usually has had a normal life with wife, children, and home?**

(a) True, (b) True, (c) False, (d) False, (e) False.

❍   **Some authors of toxicology texts have developed convenient acronyms for memorization of lists of items. Given the acronym, tell what the particular group of items have in common: (a) *WITH L.A. COPS*, (b) *SALEM TIP*, (c) *BET A CHIP*, (d) *DON'T.***

(a) Drugs causing seizures, (b) Drugs causing nystagmus, (c) Radiopaque substances, (d) Therapy for patients with altered mental status.

❍ **Some authors of toxicology texts have developed convenient acronyms for memorization of lists of items. Given the acronym, tell what the particular group of items have in common: (a) *CHAMP*, (b) *SLUGBAM*, (c) *A MUDPILE CAT*.**

(a) Additions to hydrocarbon products that cause systemic toxicity, (b) Muscarinic effects of organophosphate and carbamate insecticides, (c) Causes of anion gap metabolic acidosis.

❍ **The signs of cholinergic overdrive are remembered by the mnemonic "*SLUDGE.*" What to these letters stand for?**

Salivation, lacrimation, urination, defecation, GI hypermotility, and emesis.

❍ **A patient who is into *anti-cholinergic overdrive* often displays a set of characteristic symptoms. How does the commonly used mnemonic divide these symptoms?**

HOT as a pistol, *RED* as a beet, *BLIND* as a bat, *MAD* as a hatter, and *DRY* as a bone.

❍ **Tell whether you would expect diarrhea or constipation with each of the following intoxications: (a) Codeine, (b) Malathion, (c) *Chlorophyllum molybdites*, (d) Botulism, (e) Lead.**

(a) Constipation, (b) Diarrhea, (c) Diarrhea, (d) Constipation, (e) Constipation.

❍ **An occupational disease was commonly found in workers in the match-making industry in the early 1900s. Answer the following about this condition: (a) What chemical was the cause of this terrible condition, (b) What was the common name of this condition?**

(a) Yellow (or White) Phosphorus, (b) *"Phossy Jaw"*

❍ **What is the cause of each of the following allergic responses of the respiratory system: (a) *"Farmer's Lung,"* (b) *"Cheese Washer's Lung,"* (c) *"Bagassosis,"* (d) *"Byssinosis"*?**

(a) Thermophilic actinomycetes, (b) *Penicillium* spores, (c) Sugar cane dust, (d) Cotton, flax, or hemp dusts.

❍ **What poisonous substance is associated with each of the following conditions: (a) *"Silo Filler's Disease,"* (b) *"Hatter's Shakes,"* (c) *"Mycetism,"* (d) *"Plumbism,"* (e) *"Ginger Jake Paralysis"*?**

(a) Nitrogen oxide, Silo gas, (b) Mercury, (c) Mushrooms, (d) Lead, (e) *TOCP*, Triorthocresyl phosphate.

O   **Describe what causes the following toxicological conditions: (a) *"Hunan Hand,"* (b) *"Corn Picker's Pupil,"* (c) *"Milk Sickness,"* (d) *"Jalaproctitis"*?**

(a) Dermal exposure to *Capsicum* during cutting, (b) *Datura stramonium* in dust from corn fields during harvesting, (c) Milk contaminated by *Tremetol* from cows eating "Snakeroot," *Eupatorium rugosum*, (d) Burning discomfort on defecation after jalapeno pepper eating contests.

O   **The *"dry ice phenomenon,"* where cold seems hot, and *vice versa*, is characteristic of what type of marine poisoning?**

Ciguatera.

O   **In 1989, in St. Louis, Missouri, the death of baby Ryan Stallings from supposed ethylene glycol poisoning caused a sensation when his mother Patricia was sentenced to life in prison for intentional exposure. All charges were later dismissed when it was proven that death was due to a genetic disorder which causes a metabolic condition resulting in the body's production of toxic compounds. What is this genetic disorder called?**

"MMA," Methylmalonic acidosis.

O   **Farmhands who are chronically exposed to low levels of pesticides, show a condition characterized by nausea, weakness, and headache. What is the name of this condition?**

"Orange-picker's Flu."

O   **A individual has very low blood sugar from an excessive amount of insulin. What substance could be looked for in the body that would prove that the excessive insulin was produced by the patient or came from a source outside the body indicating suicide or homicide?**

Measure of *"C-peptide"* concentrations.

O   **A patient who has a blue color from methemoglobinemia, can be treated with a blue drug to cause a return to their natural pink color. What is the drug used?**

Methylene Blue.

O   **A patient who has been chronically exposed to arsenic will often show characteristic white transverse band markings on the nails of their hands and feet. What are these important diagnostic marks called?**

"Mees' lines."

O   **A patient who has been exposed to the very toxic compound called strychnine will exhibit a characteristic convulsion, with the body arched like a bow. What is this condition called?**

"Opisthotonus."

O   **Why is it advised that children under one year of age, should NOT be fed honey?**

Because it can contain the spores of *Clostridium botulinum*, which could lead to the development of *"Infant Botulism."*

O   **In 1966, there was a condition associated with over 1,000 people engaged in the apple-packing industry, which was traced to blue paper trays made from salvaged newsprint. What was this condition commonly called?**

"Apple Packer's Nosebleed."

O   ***"Fagopyrism"* is a disease of sheep and cattle that seems to be activated by exposure to sunlight. The ingestion of what plant is associated with this condition?**

"Buckwheat."

O   **Exposure to the fumes or mists of this chemical causes a condition known as *"mal rouge,"* which is characterized by headache, flushing, dizziness, tachypnia, and collapse. What is the causative agent?**

Calcium cyanamide.

O   **Vesicular and bullous lesions followed by depigmentation and hyper pigmentation on exposed areas of the body, came to be known as what condition on harvesters of a popular salad vegetable?**

"Celery burns."

O   **The *"Irukandji"* syndrome is thought to be due to contact with what toxic agent?**

The sting of the coelenterate *Carukia barnesi*.

O   **What condition first described in 1822 by Potissier, has become known by such common names as: *Monday Morning Fever*, *Brass Chills*, and the *Smoothers*?**

Metal Fume Fever.

O   **Intoxication by what metal may be the oldest recognized chemical toxin, being described as early as the 2nd century BC?**

Lead poisoning.

O   **Among the *Kuma* tribe of Papua New Guinea, there has been described a toxic condition described, which has become referred to as *"Kuma Madness,"* with fierce agitation. What is thought to be the cause of this condition?**

Mushrooms, which are species of the genera *Boletus* and/or *Russula*.

○   **Inhalation of what chemical in dust form, causes a condition known as *"Slag pneumonia"*?**

Thomas' slag powder, containing Calcium chloride.

○   **In the mines of the Erz mountains a lung affliction appeared in the form of *"snow mountain* pulmonary cancer." What was being mined that is thought to have lead to this condition?**

Cobalt, which was contaminated with Radium.

○   **An ashen-gray discoloration of the skin caused by small particles of this elemental sulfide, has become called *"Argyreia."* What is the elemental source of this condition?**

Silver.

○   **A condition known as *"lime-nitrogen sickness"* was caused when what substance was used as an important fertilizer?**

Calcium cyanamide.

○   **From September 1926 to August 1927, in the vicinity of Sarapoul, Russia, in a population of 506,000, there were 11,319 cases reported of intoxication with what food toxicant?**

Ergot.

○   **In 1947, Jordi reported on a condition in Swiss factory workers of necrotic skin lesions called *"powder holes."* What explosive compound was being handled which caused this condition?**

Mercuric cyanate, or *"Fulminate of mercury."*

○   **The ingestion of suarine containing fish by humans results in an allergic-like condition which includes: intense headache, gastric pain, and bronchospasm. What is this condition more commonly called?**

Scombrotoxism.

○   **In 1904, there appeared the first medical reports of a condition known as *"saddle nose deformity,"* from the use of what toxic substance?**

Cocaine.

○   **When a parent fabricates a story of disease, then poisons her child to produce symptoms; this is known as *"Munchausen Syndrome by Proxy."* It is also known as *"Polle Syndrome."* Where did it get the name *"Polle"*?**

Polle was the infant son of Baron Munchausen, who died of suspicious causes.

O   **A condition known as** *"Szechwan restaurant syndrome"* **or** *"Szechwan purpurea,"* **evidenced by small blotchy hemorrhages of the skin has been seen in some individuals. What is thought to be the component in the Chinese regional recipes which causes this condition?**

Auricularia auricula, "Black Tree Fungus."

O   **In 1886, Rayner, reported a mysterious cyanosis amongst ten infants in a maternity ward. What ultimately was proven to be the toxic cause of their condition?**

Aniline, from the ink used to mark their diapers.

O   **Some chemical substances can cause** *"parageusias."* **What happens in this condition?**

The sense of taste becomes confused, *e.g.* sweet seems salty.

O   **What substance is associated with each of the following toxic conditions: (a)** *Enriositatis,* **(b)** *Mephitism,* **(c)** *Saturnism,* **(d)** *Stibialism,* **(e)***Thebaism***?**

(a) Ethanol, (b) Carbon dioxide, (c) Lead, (d) Antimony, (e) Thebaine.

O   **In the Central African Republic, some individuals have developed a condition known as** *"Konzo."* **What toxic food substance is involved with this condition?**

Cyanide from inadequately processed *Cassava* ("Bitter Manihot").

O   **What is the name of the syndrome of unexplained rhabdomyolysis, following the consumption of certain kinds of fish, such as the "Buffalo Fish" (***Ictiobus cyprinellus***)?**

"Haff Disease."

O   **What plant is responsible for causing the condition known as** *"githagism"***?**

The Corncockle.

O   **A condition known as** *"toot poisoning,"* **is caused by the plant** *Coriaria sarmentosa.* **In what Pacific country is this plant normally found?**

New Zealand.

O   **Workers in the aircraft industry have been known to suffer from** *dural poisoning.* **What is the substance that causes this condition?**

Duraluminum (a Magnesium-Aluminum alloy).

○ **In Japan there is an intoxication known as *"esowasure-gai."* The ingestion of what type of choline containing animal causes this toxic condition?**

Shellfish of the genus *Callista.*

○ **A condition known as *"bongkrek intoxication"* or *"tempeh poisoning,"* is caused by the ingestion of a dish made from the faulty fermentation of molds from copra press cake. In what Asian country is the dish *bongkrek* popular?**

Java.

○ **Eating excessive amounts of the bean, *Pitecolobium lobatum*, can cause a condition exhibiting the signs of pain in the renal region, dysuria, and anuria. What is this condition called?**

"Djenkol poisoning."

EPIDEMICS AND DISASTERS

○   In a famous hotel fire in 1980, 79 of 94 people died who were far removed from the actual flames. Their deaths being due to inhalation of toxic smoke and fumes. What was the name of the hotel which burned?

The *MGM Grand Hotel.*

○   On December 7, 1917, the French freighter *"Mont Blanc"* collided with another ship and its cargo of *TNT*, picric acid, and benzene exploded. The fatalities numbered between 2,000 to 4,000, with some 8,000 people injured, and 4 square kilometers of the city center leveled. In what city's harbor did this terrible chemical disaster occur?

Halifax, Nova Scotia, Canada.

○   The date was 1951, when in Atlanta, Georgia, a mass poisoning occurred from bootleg whiskey, that resulted in over 300 cases of poisoning and at least 41 deaths. The 60 gallons of whiskey were contaminated with up to 35% of what toxic chemical?

Methanol.

○   In 1988, it was revealed that over 44 patients were murdered in the largest number of killings ever known in a European hospital, when nurses used insulin and night-time sedatives, to do away with nuisance cases. In what city and country did these killings occur?

Vienna, Austria.

○   In February 1990, there was a 120 country recall of some 160 million bottles of Perrier® water due to possible contamination with what toxic chemical, through dirty filters?

Benzene.

○   What countries, IN ORDER, would you travel to, if you wanted to take a chartered tour of sites of famous toxicological disasters, and your flight plan went from *Minamata Bay* to *Chernobyl* to *Bhopal* to *Seveso*?

Japan – Soviet Union – India – Italy.

○   In 1978, with wide media attention, the residents of an area in New York State were evacuated from their homes because of the grave and imminent peril resulting from the presence of approximately 20,000 tons of toxic waste dumped by the *Hooker Chemical and Plastics Company*. By what name was this residential area known?

"Love Canal."

O   In the fall of 1987, a number of people who ate the cultivated "Blue Mussel" (*Mytilis edulus*), became ill with some cases ending in fatality. The agent responsible for the outbreak was determined to be Demoic acid, a naturally occurring amino acid. On what island did this outbreak occur?

Prince Edward Island, Canada.

O   A massive French recall of the 1991 edition of the best selling European dictionary *Petit Larousse en Coulerus*, had to be undertaken when a mistake was found on page 203, which could have lead to toxicological consequences. What was the error?

Some illustrations of mushrooms had been incorrectly coded, indicating that the very toxic *Amanita phalloides*, *Amanita virosa*, and *Cortinarius orellannus*, were harmless.

O   An epidemic in Japan in 1968, caused infants exposed *in utero* to be born with swollen eyelids, mental retardation, and a peculiar skin discoloration known as *"cola babies."* What contaminant of rice bran oil was the cause of this condition?

PCB, Polychlorinated biphenyl.

O   In 1776, a physician named Sir John Baker, solved a condition in England which was known as *"The Devonshire Colic."* What was the cause of this condition which had been associated with the production of cider in Devonshire?

He determined that the use of lead in sealing the cider presses, resulted in leaching of lead by the acidic cider.

O   Concerns were high when a January 1992 storm off Cape May, New Jersey, caused 441 barrels of what toxic compound to fall off the freighter *"Santa Clara I,"* onto the floor of the Atlantic Ocean?

Arsenic trioxide.

O   What poisonous creature was imported into Australia in 1934 to prey upon beetles, and instead, turned into an environmental folly?

The "Caine Toad," *Bufo marinus*.

O   On November 28, 1942, in the city of Boston, Massachusetts, 490 people died from the direct result of flames or the toxic fumes from burning plastics. At the time this was the second deadliest building fire in the nation's history. In what famous supper club did this toxic disaster occur?

"The Coconut Grove."

○ In 1933, in the state of California, a bag of poisoned barley, which was intended for squirrel eradication, was stolen. The grain was used to make tortillas. Of the 31 consumers, 20 became ill, of which 14 were hospitalized, and of which 7 died. What was the toxic agent?

Thallium.

○ One of the most serious accidental mass exposures occurred in the 1940s, when in a State hospital, 261 patients, of which 47 (18%) died, were given what compound in the belief that it was powdered milk?

Sodium fluoride.

○ In May 1988, a series of massive explosions in what city demolished one of only two plants producing ammonium perchlorate for the U.S. space shuttles and *MX* missiles.

Henderson, Nevada.

○ From December 3-5, 1930, meteorologic conditions in the *Meuse River Valley* promoted the concentration of factory smoke that resulted in 65 deaths. This was the first significant industrial air pollution disaster. Near what city, and in what country did this event occur?

Liege, Belgium.

○ In France in 1952, 234 babies became ill and 69 died when they were dusted with a baby powder that, due to a labeling error, contained what toxic substance?

Arsenic.

○ In October 1980, a "blow out" on board the oil rig *"Ron Tapmeyer"* produced a cloud of poison gas in which 8 men suffocated and another 19 were affected. What was the toxic gas produced?

Hydrogen sulfide.

○ In 1937, the new wonder drug *sulfanilamide* was introduced as an elixir. The vehicle for this elixir was thought to be safe but resulted in the deaths of 76 people. What chemical served as this toxic vehicle?

Diethylene glycol.

○ A major incident of poisoning occurred in Morocco in 1959, affecting 10,000 people who had eaten food cooked in olive oil adulterated with contaminated lubricating oil containing what toxic compound?

TOCP, Tri-*o*-cresyl-phosphate.

❍   In the 1970s, there was a problem in the U.S. when children came into contact with the mutagen *tris* (2,3-dibromopropyl)phosphate, commonly called *"Tris."* How did they come into contact with this compound.

It was a flame retardant used in children's sleepwear.

❍   In the 1970s, the production of what insecticidal compound in Hopewell, Virginia, resulted in the discharge of about 53,000 kilograms of this compound into the James River, through the city sewage system.

Kepone.

❍   In 1968, several hundred people in Japan became ill from what was called *"Yusho"* or *"rice oil disease."* What was the toxic contaminant which was found in a concentration as high as 3,000 *ppm*?

PCB, polychlorinated biphenyls.

❍   A large poisoning incident hit this island county in 1976, when 17 deaths (22%) were recorded from 79 people who had ingested flour which had been contaminated with the insecticide parathion. Where did this happen?

Jamaica.

❍   From 1957-61, there was marketed in the United States a sedative and hypnotic drug which left in its international wake over 10,000 deformed infants. This drug which is considered a prototype teratogen in man, is known by what name?

Thalidomide, (*alpha*-phthalmidoglutarimide).

❍   December 1984, 45 metric tons of what chemical escaped from a pesticide plant in Bhopal, India, which killed an estimated 2,500 people?

Methyl isocyanate.

❍   In 1929, a fire at the *Cleveland Clinic,* killed 97 workers immediately from Carbon monoxide and Hydrogen cyanide intoxication, plus 26 delayed fatalities from fumes of Nitrous oxides. What was the specific source for these toxic fumes?

The burning of 50,000 nitro-cellulose X-ray films.

❍   In May 1981, an epidemic occurred in Spain, affecting more than 20,000 persons, and causing more than 11,000 hospital admissions, and 340 deaths. This disease is now known as the *"toxic oil syndrome."* The cause of the condition was attributed to ingestion of an industrial oil that had been marketed as olive oil. What was the name of this industrial oil?

Rapeseed Oil - which was denatured with 2% aniline.

❍ It is now known that the cause of a disease called *"Pa Ping"* (in the Szechnen area of China) which is characterized by transient paralysis, is due to salt which was heavily contaminated with what toxic compound?

Barium chloride.

❍ On April 26, 1986, reactor #4, released an estimated 50 million curies of radiation into the environment from what nuclear plant?

Chernobyl, Soviet Union.

❍ It has been estimated that in 1988, some 360 kilograms of mercury were released into the atmosphere in Sweden. One scientist proposed reducing the release by placing a container of Selenium on the sources, to trap emitted Mercury vapors as Mercury selenide crystals. What was the unusual source of this mercury release?

It was vaporized from dental amalgams, in crematoria.

❍ In 1991, 135 people became ill after eating beef liver from animals treated with a veterinary drug called *Clenbuterol*, which had been used to increase muscle development. In what country did this epidemic occur?

Spain.

❍ What United States company was sued by the Indian government after the poisoning of thousands of people in 1984?

Union Carbide.

❍ When one hears the name *Times Beach*, Missouri, what toxicological contamination in 1983, should come to mind?

The infamous spread of dioxin from the use of waste oil sprayed on roads to keep down dust.

❍ In the summer of 1992, a train tank car carrying Benzene spilled into the *Nemadji River*, causing a toxic cloud to form, which forced 50,000 residents to flee their homes. What was the name of the unfortunate city in Minnesota that saw this disaster?

Duluth.

❍ In 1988, while working in Charleston, at the *Olin Chemical* plant, fifty construction workers were exposed to hot mercury vapor while cutting a piping system. This incident, which is to date the worst industrial exposure to mercury in United States history, occurred in what state?

Tennessee.

❍   **In the 1960s, in Great Britain, 100,000 turkeys perished from a mysterious disease known as *"Turkey X Disease."* The cause of death was eventually traced back to their feed which consisted of moldy Brazilian peanut meal. This investigation lead to the discovery of what toxic group of compounds?**

Aflatoxins. *Aflatoxin B1,* is one of the most powerful carcinogenic compounds known today, being about 75 times as powerful as dimethylnitrosamine.

❍   **In July 1976, there occurred a toxicological disaster known as the *"Seveso Incident,"* which covered some 733 acres. Answer the following about this chemical disaster: (a) In what country did this disaster occur?, (b) What chemical was released into the environment?, (c) What quantity by weight was estimated to have been released?**

(a) Italy, (b) *TCDD*, 2,3,7,8-tetrachlorodibenzo-p-dioxin, (c) 4 lbs.

❍   **In 1968, there occurred the famous *"Skull Valley Incident,"* of environmental contamination by a toxic agent. Answer the following about this incident: (a) In what State of the United States did this event occur? (b) What substance leaked from a spray tank? (c) Who or what were the victims of this contamination?**

(a) Utah, (b) The nerve gas agent *"VX,"* release of ~20 lbs., (c) Herds of sheep, with about 6,000 deaths.

❍   **In 1991 another case of product tampering struck in the United States. Answer the following about this incident: (a) What was the contaminant?, (b) What product was involved?, (c) Who was the manufacturer of the product?, (d) What State was the site of the tampering?**

(a) Cyanide, (b) Sudafed 12-Hour capsules, (c) Burroughs Welcome, (d) Washington.

❍   **On September 13, 1986, some youths playing in an abandoned building in the South American town of Goiania, found a 300 lb. lead capsule. They took it home and broke it open with a hammer, to find it contained a blue powder that glowed in the dark. Handling of the powder contaminated 249 people, of which the four who died had to be buried in two feet of concrete as they would be radioactive for 200 years. Answer the following about this incident: (a) In what country did this amazing event occur? (b) What was the toxic contents of the container?**

(a) Brazil, (b) Cesium-*137.*

❍   **On November 8, 1989, a series of 16 cases of an unusual syndrome were reported by the *CDC* involving an *OTC* product being used for insomnia and pre-menstrual symptoms. The syndrome manifest by an increased presence of a certain kind of white blood cells and muscle swelling and weakness, resulted in more than 2,000 reported cases, 19 deaths, and withdrawal of the product from the market by the *FDA*. Answer the following about this syndrome: (a) Name the syndrome, (b) Name the product, (c) Name the State where the first cases were** discovered, **(d) Name the country where the manufacturer was located, (e) Name the company which manufactured the agent.**

(a) "Eosinophilia-Myalgia-Syndrome" (*EMS*), (b) The amino acid L-tryptophan, (c) New Mexico, (d) Japan, (e) *Shona Denka*.

❍   **In November 1986, there occurred in Europe an environmental contaminations which has come to be known as the *"Schweizerhalle"* accident. Answer the following about this catastrophe: (a) In what city did this occur? (b) What was the name of the company involved? (c) What was the initiating cause of the accident? (d) What chemical had the most serious environmental impact? (e) What waterway was ecologically damaged?**

(a) Basel, Switzerland, (b) Sandoz, (c) A fire, the 10,000 m^3 of extinguishing water carried 30,000, tons of chemicals in the runoff, (d) Mercury compounds, 150 kilograms, (e) Rhine river.

❍   **In 1971, a toxicological event caused 6,530 people to be hospitalized for mercury toxicity, with 459 deaths resulting. Answer the following about this event: (a) What was the toxic agent? (b) How did the toxic agent enter the victim's system? (c) In what country did this tragedy occur?**

(a) Organic mercurial fungicide, (b) When seed grain was used for food, (c) Iraq.

❍   **In the 1980s, a tragedy occurred in the United States, when some capsules of *Tylenol*® were tampered with to contain cyanide. Answer the following about this terrible event: (a) In what city did this incident occur? (b) In what year did this happen? (c) How many known victims died in this incident? (d) Who was eventually identified as the actual tamperer?**

(a) Chicago, Illinois, (b) 1982, (c) 7, (d) To date, the tamperer has never been found.

❍   **A massive contamination of the population living in the *Jintsu River Valley*, near the city of *Fuchu*, occurre through dietary exposure to a toxic substance. Answer the following about this incident: (a) In what country did this occur?, (b) The victims were afflicted by what was called *"itai, itai"* disease. What is the English equivalent to the name of this condition?, (c) The ingestion of what toxic substance was the cause of this condition?, (d) What was the attributed source of this contamination?**

(a) Japan, (b) *"Ouch, ouch,"* because of the painful osteomalacia, (c) Cadmium, (d) Irrigated rice contaminated from an upstream mine producing Lead, Zinc, and Cadmium.

❍   **In his famous story *"Eleven Blue Men,"* author Berton Roueche, relates the epidemiological detective work that sent in to determining the cause of a 1944 incident in which a compound was erroneously added, instead of salt, to a cafeteria's oatmeal, producing massive symptoms. Answer the following about this incident: (a) What was the toxic condition caused by the chemical? (b) What** compound was the cause of the condition? (c) What antidote would be used to treat this condition?

(a) Methemoglobinemia, (b) Sodium nitrate, *"Saltpeter,"* (c) Methylene Blue.

○   The year 1973, saw in the United States, a large scale agricultural disaster when *Firemaster FF-1®*, a fire retardant was accidentally added to livestock feed, instead of *Nutrimaster®* (Magnesium oxide). Up to 97% of the general population of one of the states was felt to be contaminated through the food chain. Answer the following about this disaster: (a) What was the toxic chemical involved?, (b) In what state did this tragedy occur?

(a) Polybrominated biphenyls, or *PBB*, (b) Michigan.

○   In the United States, in October 1994, there was a national recall of *Salmonella enteriditis* contaminated ice cream products from a manufacturer located in Marshall, Minnesota. What was the name of this popular home-delivered ice cream?

Schwan's.

○   The most famous case of poisoning with this toxic compound occurred at the *Oregon State Hospital* in 1943, when workers accidentally mixed 11 pounds of this salt with 10 gallons of scrambled eggs, killing 47 of the 263 persons who ingested the contaminated food. What was the toxic salt?

Sodium fluoride.

○   In 1944, more than 500 persons died from Carbon monoxide exposure, when their train was stalled in a tunnel.   Where did this disaster take place?

Salerno, Italy.

○   In 1990, in the Bronx, New York, 87 people died from the inhalation of toxic fumes when their unlicenced club caught fire. What was the name of this unfortunate party place?

"Happy Land Social Club."

○   In May, 1928, some tanks of gas on the *Hofe Canal*, Hamburg, Germany, leaked and the fumes resulted in multiple deaths from the poison. What chemical was contained in the tanks?

Phosgene.

○   In December 1994, more than 50 deaths were reported in an African country after some residents consumed homemade whisky known as *"kaporroto,"* which had been adulterated with Methanol. In what country did this tragedy occur?

Luanda, Angola.

○   **In 1985, in the state of California, there was an acute outbreak of toxicological significance, when the insecticide *Aldicarb* was found to have contaminated what popular food?**

Watermelons.

○   **In June 1994, a toxic chemical seeped through the open windows of homes in the Japanese city of Matsumoto, killing 8 people, and seriously poisoning 200 inhabitants. What was this toxic gas?**

The nerve gas *Sarin*.

○   **In September 1918, in the village of *Bierzglin*, near *Poznan*, Poland, 31 children died within a few days after eating a meal made with what toxic substance?**

Mushrooms, *Amanita phalloides.*

○   **In 1990, in a village near Beijing, China, 176 people suffered neurological symptoms from flour that had been contaminated at the local mill, with leaking lubricating oil. What was the toxic chemical component?**

Tricresyl phosphate, *TCP.*

○   **During the months of May and June 1985, unpasteurized orange juice contaminated with the *Salmonella* organism sickened 63 visitors to what popular American tourist spot?**

Disney World, Orlando, Florida.

○   **In 1945, 85 British soldier in India, were poisoned by a toxic contaminant in their flour. What was the contaminant?**

Barium carbonate.

○   **In November 1993, 188 people were admitted to the hospital after consuming the meat of a single shark (*Carcharhinus leucas*). Of the 200 poisoned inhabitants, the mortality rate was nearly 30%. On what island country did this tragic ciguatoxic event occur?**

Manakara, Madagascar.

○   **If one turned on the radio to *CBS*, on October 30, 1938, one might have heard reports of a war being waged that included amongst its weapons, a *"poisonous black smoke"* that was killing hundreds of innocent civilians. What war was being described?**

"The War of the Worlds," by *The Mercury Theater On the Air.*

○   **In England, in the 1850s, there was an infamous incident called *"The Bradford Lozenge Poisoning."* What was the cause of this toxicological disaster?**

A cask of white arsenic was mistakenly added to the ingredients of a confectioner's peppermints.

❍   **In Loughton, Essex, England in 1877-78, there occurred a disaster when a grocer supposedly substituted white arsenic for starch in baby powder. The resultant baby powder which was at least 25% arsenic, resulted in 28 cases, including 13 fatalities, of poisoning in infants. What was this incident called?**

"The Violet Powder Case."

❍   **In Japan, near *Lake Hamana*, an outbreak of *"asai"* poisoning had a mortality rate of 35%. What was the cause of this epidemic?**

Ingestion of short-necked clams, *Venerupin Shellfish Poisoning.*

❍   **The worst subway disaster in history occurred in *Baku*, when over 300 people died from Carbon monoxide and other toxic fumes formed when a subway car caught fire. In what country did this tragedy occur?**

Azerbaijan.

❍   **The day April 11, 1996, saw a fire in a major German airport, in which 16 people died from the inhalation of toxic fumes. In which city did this tragedy occur?**

Dusseldorf.

❍   **During a three month period, in 1996, 21 people died in this European region, after purchasing in street markets, local brandies and foreign liquors which were created from water, artificial coloring, and Methanol. In what European geographic area did this terrible toxic "rip-off" occur?**

Serbia.

❍   **It was announced in 1996, that some bottles of *OTC* antipyretic medications (*Afebril* and *Valodon*), had been contaminated with Ethylene glycol. The intoxications resulted in the deaths of at least 55 children. In what Carribean country did this toxic disaster occur?**

Haiti.

❍   **On December 5, 1952, a major European city suffered a massive *"killer smog"* air pollution disaster that took the lives of over 4,000 people. What city suffered such a disaster?**

London, England.

❍   **The world's largest outbreak of arsenic poisoning started 30 years ago with engineers digging new wells to irrigate rice crops. The contaminated water, with up to 10 mg/Liter of arsenic, is estimated to have poisoned at least 200,000 people. In what country is this disaster taking place?**

West Bengal.

○   **In 1988, an environmental incident occurred in Cornwall, England, when 20 tons of a substance were accidentally poured into the *South West Water's Lowermoor* treatment works. What substance was involved in what became known as the *"Camelford Water Poisoning Incident"*?**

Aluminum sulphate.

○   **In January 1986, a tragedy struck when 14 patients died in an Asian hospital when they were given glycerol, which had been contaminated with Diethylene glycol. In what city and country did this toxic tragedy occur?**

Bombay, India.

○   **Around 1946, 80 officers and men of the Swiss army were poisoned when they ate cheese fritters, which had been fried in oil issued as an anti-rust fluid. What was the toxic ingredient?**

TOCP, Tri-ortho-cresyl-phosphate.

○   **In 1976, the Hudson River in New York State was inadvertently contaminated with what toxic substance?**

PCB, Polychlorinated biphenyl.

○   **As early as 1895, a high incidence of bladder tumors were described in German workers involved in the production of what colorful materials?**

Dyes.

○   **In 1975, the substance Malathion was being utilized for the control of malaria. Of the 7,500 individuals spraying, 2,800 became ill, and 5 died from the isomerization product iso-malathion. In what Asian country did this epidemic occur?**

Pakistan.

○   **In January 1997, 32 people were killed by a deadly brew of homemade liquor in the Asian city of *Hyderabad*. In what Islamic country did this disaster occur?**

Pakistan.

○   **In 1997, there was an outbreak of toxic exposures the face creams *"Crema de Belleza"* and *"Nutrapiel,"* manufactured in Mexico, which contained what toxic metallic substance?**

Mercury.

❍   Because of the demand by wealthy diners for *"Groupers"* and *"Humphead Wrasses,"* the coral reefs of Indonesia and the Philippines are being decimated by the use of what toxic substance to obtain these culinary delights?

Sodium cyanide.

❍   In 1995, global worries began concerning pollution of the world's oceans by what radioactive military sources?

Mishaps at sea which resulted in the loss, from submarines, of 19 reactors and at least 43 nuclear weapons.

❍   In 1910, the world was in a panic because the earth was going to pass through what the tail of what cosmic event, which was supposed to be rich with toxic cyanogen.

"Halley's Comet."

❍   During March, 1997, 14 Massachusetts teenagers at a *"Boys and Girls Club"* dance, were lucky to survive, after taking large amounts of what prescription drug trying to get high?

Baclofen.

❍   In 1956, in Brazil, there began a toxicological disaster when what group of toxic animals entered the natural fauna?

"Africanized Honey Bees."

❍   In April 1984, New Hampshire public health officials traced an outbreak of acute diarrhea among numerous children to what popular treat they were consuming?

Dietetic candies containing Sorbitol.

❍   In 1977, an unusually high incidence of what condition was experienced by *Lathrop*, California workers who were exposed during the production of a nematocide, to Dibromochloro-propane (*DBCP*)?

Sterility amongst male workers.

❍   In April 1996, three cases of an unusual food borne poison were reported in San Diego, California, which was attributed to the consumption of a food product imported by a Japanese traveler, which was undeclared at customs?

Tetrodotoxin, from prepackaged *Fugu* fish.

❍   In 1997, the *Tottenville* branch of the *New York Public Library* was closed shortly after renovation because many people were becoming ill from what toxic source?

Growing in damp areas, the fungus *Stachybotrys atra*, was releasing toxic spores, resulting in the *"Sick Building Syndrome"* .

○ **On April 13, 1994, an 18-wheeler truck carrying 22 tons of a pesticide crashed and burned. Five thousand people were evacuated from the surrounding area, and 389 calls were made to the local Poison Center in the first 24 hours. Answer the following about this incident: (a) In what city this incident occur, (b) What pesticide was involved?**

(a) Balch Springs, Texas, (b) Aldicarb.

○ **In 1994, an adulteration of a cooking condiment sent one nation reeling. To boost profits, unethical dealers cut a spice with toxic paint, which ultimately resulted in 108 cases of lead poisoning. Answer the following about this incident: (a) In what European country did this event occur, (b) What national spice was so adulterated?**

(a) Hungary, (b) Paprika.

○ **In June, 1971, a massive nationwide food recall was created when a soup manufacturer was found to have sold cans of product which contained deadly botulinus toxin, because their cans had been inadequately heat treated, and ultimately resulted in at least one consumer's death. The negative financial impact of the recall ultimately lead to the closure of the 100 year old firm. Answer the following about this incident: (a) What was the name of the soup's manufacturer, (b) What was the type of soup that was recalled, (c) In what city and state was this manufacturer located?**

(a) *Bon Vivant, Inc.*, (b) *"Vichyssoise Soup,"* (c) Newark, New Jersey.

○ **On February 20, 1995, there was a chemical disaster on a mass transit system in a major Asian city. Answer the following about this incident: (a) In what city did this disaster occur? (b) What group was the offender? (c) Who was the group's leader? (d) What chemical was supposedly used?**

(a) Tokyo, Japan, (b) *Aum Shiniri* ("Supreme Truth"), (c) Shoko Ashahari, (d) Sarin, nerve gas.

○ **August, 1981, saw the deaths of 177 (24%) of 741 infant pediatric cases of a hemorrhagic syndrome, which was traced to talcum powder which had been contaminated with 1.7%-6.5% warfarin. In what Asian City and country did this toxic tragedy occur?**

Ho Chi Minh City, Vietnam.

○ **On January 13, 1998, thirty *Texarkana* residents were evacuated from their homes, after contamination occurred when youths stole a chemical from am abandoned Neon plant. Some youths even smoked cigarettes which had been dipped into this toxic substance. What was the substance that caused this crisis?**

Mercury.

❍   **In January 1998, there was a massive recall of *Hostess*® snack goodies made in the plant at Schiller Park, Illinois. What was the atmospheric contaminant during the production process?**

Asbestos.

❍   **In 1998, one of the world's largest outbreaks of poisoning from Methanol, with over 44 deaths, and over 120 hospitalizations, took place in an Asian country. Answer the following about this incident: (a) In what country did this disaster take place? (b) What was identified as the source of the poisoning?**

(a) Cambodia, (b) An adulterated locally produced wine with herbs and plants.

❍   **In 1998, the United States *Consumer Products Safety Commission* recalled 2,500 Warner Brothers *"Tweety Water Timer Game Key Rings,"* due to a toxic ingredient in the toy's formulation. What was the toxic ingredient?**

Ethylene glycol.

❍   **In 1984, 23 Baltic fisherman suffered toxic effects from what substance caught in their nets?**

"Mustard Gas" ammunition, from World War II.

GEOGRAPHY

○ **In the 1950s, a tragedy struck certain members of the Japanese population, due to contamination of offshore fishing waters with mercury containing compounds. What is the common name of this toxicological condition?**

Minamata Disease.

○ **The *Jivaro* Indians of Ecuador, cover their blow-gun darts with a plant poison which causes skeletal muscle paralysis. This plant chemical has also found use in critical care medicine. What is the name of the active ingredient of this plant?**

Curare.

○ **What Latin American country expelled three United States diplomats in 1983, for allegedly plotting to poison its defense minister?**

Nicaragua.

○ **In Soviet Russia, it is known as the *"Karakurt,"* in the Antilles as *"Coulrouge, 24 horas,"* in Australia as the *"Katipo."* By what common name is this spider better known in the United States?**

"Black Widow," or *"Hour-glass Spider."*

○ **On November 18, 1978, a tragedy occurred involving many deaths from cyanide. Where did this event, which lead to the deaths of over 900 people, occur?**

People's Temple commune, Jonestown, Guyana.

○ **After *World War II*, it was important that a large number of hedgehogs were released in order to develop the Black Sea coast of Bulgaria and the Adriatic coast of Yugoslavia as tourist areas. Why was this?**

To wipe out the venomous snakes indigenous to these regions. The hedgehog can be bitten without much endangerment to its life, and is thus the natural enemy of these snakes.

○ **If you sailed to an island and joined a native ceremony, where participants used the powdered roots of the "kava-kava" (*Piper methysticum*), to prepare a hypnotic drink, in which area of the world's oceans would you be sailing?**

The South Pacific. Mainly the islands of *Fiji*, *Tonga*, and *Samoa*.

○   **In the proposed construction of a sea level canal through Panama, what is a toxicological concern about the possible consequences of the canal's presence?**

The migration of sea snakes, or the *"Crown of Thorns"* starfish, from the Pacific Ocean to the Atlantic Ocean.

○   **While serving as United States Ambassador to Italy in the 1950s, Clare Booth Luce suffered intoxication from paint chips falling into her food from the ceiling of our embassy in Rome. What substance was responsible for her toxic symptoms?**

Arsenic.

○   **The venomous snake called the true *"Fer de Lance"* (*Bothrops lanceolatus*), can be found only on a single island in the world. What is the name of this island habitat?**

The French West Indian island of *Martinique*.

○   **In what two oceans will one find most of the world's sea snakes?**

Pacific Ocean and Indian Ocean.

○   **In the roaring 1920s, this American city was so crime ridden that the Attorney General proclaimed it *"the poison spot of the nation."* What city got this verbal black eye?**

St. Paul, Minnesota.

○   **Which North American nation has a rattlesnake on it's flag?**

Mexico.

○   **An anthropologist listens as natives of a desert area describe their use of a natural poison they call "Nga," obtained from the "leaf beetle" (*Diamphidia simplex*), to poison their hunting arrows. In what great southern desert area would this conversation be taking place?**

Kalahari Desert, Africa.

○   **Black Widow spiders can be found widely distributed around the world, but there is one state in the United States, in which these spiders are thought NOT to be found native. Which state is it?**

Alaska.

○   **On August 21, 1986, residents experienced a catastrophic event when *Lake Nyos* suddenly belched a massive amount of Carbon dioxide gas, which proved lethal to a distance of 10 kilometers. Approximately 1,700 people and 3,000 cattle died from asphyxiation, when this disaster occurred in what country?**

Cameroon, West Africa.

○ **During the month of August, 1991, six members of the militant *"Liberation Tigers of Tamil Eelam,"* committed suicide by drinking cyanide, to avoid capture as the police closed in. In what country did this take place?**

India.

○ **What American state hosts an annual festival named after the venomous fire ant?**

Texas.

○ **The national emblem of what country depicts an eagle holding a rattlesnake in its mouth?**

Mexico.

○ **One-half of the world's mercury is supplied by what two European nations?**

Italy and Spain.

○ **For centuries, whalers from what country, tipped their harpoons with a paste made from the crushed seeds of *Aconitum japonicum*?**

Japan.

○ **A pint of saturated salt water contains approximately 169 grams, or 2,900 milliequivalents, of NaCl. But, drinking a pint of this solution was a traditional method of suicide in what Asian country?**

China.

○ **It you were in the village of *Cocullo* in the *Abruzzi* mountains of Italy, on the 4th of August, you would be able to watch a religious festival to *Saint Dominic*, which utilizes some toxic objects. What would you see carried in the festival procession?**

Snakes, both venomous and nonvenomous.

○ **Four plants or flowers are used to symbolize the countries of Great Britain. Which of them, if any, are toxic?**

None! They are: *rose* (England), *leek* (Wales), *thistle* (Scotland) and *shamrock* (Ireland).

○ **In what island country do more people die of snakebite each year than in any other comparable area of the world, with an annual death rate of approximately 800 people?**

Sri Lanka.

○   **Which country in the Western hemisphere, is thought to represent the world's richest area in diversity and use of hallucinogens in aboriginal societies?**

Mexico.

○   **In the 1920s, a radium dial factory in this Midwest town, in the United States, lead to contamination of the city environment, to which many cancers in the local inhabitants have been attributed, leading to the nickname *"Radium City."* Name the city and state of this calamity?**

Ottawa, Illinois.

○   **What Southern state introduced the lethal injection as a form of execution in 1982?**

Texas.

○   **If, while visiting Samoa, you were served toxic*"Matamulu,"* what would you be eating?**

A raw sea anemone, *Rhodactis howesii*, the eating of which can cause respiratory failure.

○   **If you were drinking in Southeast Asia, and were offered a glass of *"Mamushi Whiskey,"* would the toxicologically-related added component be: animal, vegetable, or mineral?**

Animal, the *"Mamushi"* snake, *Agkistrodon*.

○   **From early times people of what country are said to have used gold leaf for suicidal purposes, and when a high official put an end to his life it was officially announced that he had *"taken gold leaf"*?**

China.

○   **If you were visiting amongst the *Cholo* Indian tribe, and they were describing a hunting poison which they had used for centuries, which they called *"kong-KWAY PAH."* What would they be describing?**

The *"Kokoi Arrow Poison Frog,"* of Columbia, a source of homobatrachotoxin.

○   **One of the most important research centers in the world for venoms is the *Instituto Butantan*. Where is it located?**

Sao Paulo, Brazil.

○   **What state in the United States has a rattlesnake as part of the official State Seal?**

New Mexico.

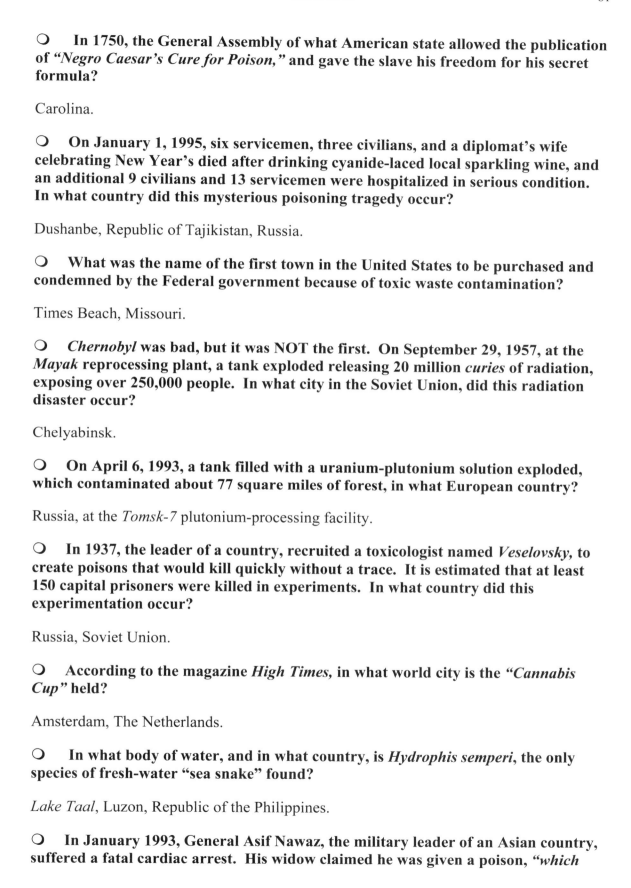

O   **In 1750, the General Assembly of what American state allowed the publication of *"Negro Caesar's Cure for Poison,"* and gave the slave his freedom for his secret formula?**

Carolina.

O   **On January 1, 1995, six servicemen, three civilians, and a diplomat's wife celebrating New Year's died after drinking cyanide-laced local sparkling wine, and an additional 9 civilians and 13 servicemen were hospitalized in serious condition. In what country did this mysterious poisoning tragedy occur?**

Dushanbe, Republic of Tajikistan, Russia.

O   **What was the name of the first town in the United States to be purchased and condemned by the Federal government because of toxic waste contamination?**

Times Beach, Missouri.

O   ***Chernobyl* was bad, but it was NOT the first. On September 29, 1957, at the *Mayak* reprocessing plant, a tank exploded releasing 20 million *curies* of radiation, exposing over 250,000 people. In what city in the Soviet Union, did this radiation disaster occur?**

Chelyabinsk.

O   **On April 6, 1993, a tank filled with a uranium-plutonium solution exploded, which contaminated about 77 square miles of forest, in what European country?**

Russia, at the *Tomsk-7* plutonium-processing facility.

O   **In 1937, the leader of a country, recruited a toxicologist named *Veselovsky*, to create poisons that would kill quickly without a trace. It is estimated that at least 150 capital prisoners were killed in experiments. In what country did this experimentation occur?**

Russia, Soviet Union.

O   **According to the magazine *High Times,* in what world city is the *"Cannabis Cup"* held?**

Amsterdam, The Netherlands.

O   **In what body of water, and in what country, is *Hydrophis semperi*, the only species of fresh-water "sea snake" found?**

Lake Taal, Luzon, Republic of the Philippines.

O   **In January 1993, General Asif Nawaz, the military leader of an Asian country, suffered a fatal cardiac arrest. His widow claimed he was given a poison, *"which*** *clogs the veins and leads to death by heart attack."* **Of what country was this man the leader?**

Pakistan.

❍ **What country has the largest selection of indigenous toxic marine and land animals?**

Australia.

❍ **Optic and peripheral neuropathies, thought to be due to the presence of some toxic substance in the diet, plagued the inhabitants of what island nation in the 1980s and 1990s?**

Cuba.

❍ **In 1992, a young man named Chris McCandless walked into the woods determined to survive and gain the wilderness experience. He died alone from *"Swainsonine"* alkaloidal poisoning, as a result of eating the seed pods of the "Wild Potato" (*Hedysarum alpinum*), and his tragic ordeal was detailed in the book *Into the Wild*, by Jon Krakauer. In what U.S. state did he succumb from his tragic error?**

Alaska.

❍ **During the 15ᵗʰ and 16ᵗʰ centuries Italy was know by what name because of the widespread reputation it had for the land of many poisoners?**

"Venenosa Italia."

❍ **In which world country is it estimated that 200,00 people are bitten by venomous snakes each year, with 10,000-15,000 deaths?**

India.

❍ **In which country is toad venom collected, dried, and used for treating heart disease, as a product called *"Ch'an Su"*?**

China.

❍ **In which country of the world is it estimated that the victim has the greatest chance of dying from the bite of a venomous snake?**

Burma.

❍ **In 1994, it was theorized that explorers Robert O'Hara and William John Wills, who in 1860-61, led a famous expedition across this land mass, may have died due to excessive thiminase intake and consequent beriberi. It was thought that the excessive thimainase source may have been freshwater mussels and *"Nardoo"* fern, *Marsilea drummondii*. What land mass were these men exploring?**

Australia.

O   **Where did host country opponents of the 1996 *"Miss World"* contest, threaten, in protest, to commit suicide with Cyanide on the final day of the competition?**

India.

O   **The English poet Samuel Butler (1835-1902) once penned a couplet: *"The Prince of Cambay's daily food – Is asp and basilik and toad, — Which makes him have so strong a breath — Each night he stinks a queen to death."* In what Asian country would one find the Prince of Cambay?**

India.

O   **While traveling in France, you receive a gift of *"wild"* mushrooms to prepare for dinner. However, in this country one can obtain assistance from what health professional resource?**

Local retail pharmacists will assist in identification, for a fee.

O   **Name the Asian country where police have been given permission to use poisonous snakes against rioters?**

Indonesia.

O   **In September 1997, the government of Israel was embarrassed from their bungled assassination attempt on *Hamas* leader Khalid Mashaal, by brushing poison on his skin. In what city and country, did this assassination attempt occur?**

Aman, Jordan.

O   **In 1995, Prince Thitibhand Yugala, collapsed after drinking a cup of coffee in his Asian palace. It was suspected that his wife had placed a pesticide in the drink to eliminate him. In what country did this occur?**

Thailand.

O   **In January 1998, 19 members of a doomsday cult were detained after they tried to commit suicide for a second time. The cult members, mostly German, believed that a spaceship would rescue their souls from the summit of the *Teide* volcano on this island. Where did this event transpire?**

Tenerife, Canary Islands.

O   **List the continents (Africa, Americas, Asia, Australia, and Europe) in order from most to least, as far as the number of types of dangerous snakes they contain.**

Asia > Americas > Africa > Australia > Europe.

❍   **The first riot control agent to be used was Ethyl bromoacetate when, in 1912, it was used in what major European city?**

Paris, France.

HISTORY: ANCIENT

○   In the Egyptian manuscript *Papyrus Ebers* there is mention of *"speak not the name of I.A.O. under the penalty of the peach."* To what toxic chemical is this thought to refer?

Cyanogenic glycosides, or Cyanide.

○   Socrates, condemned by the Athenian State, was executed by means of an extract of a toxic plant. What plant was supposedly used?

"Poison Hemlock," *Conium maculatum.*

AA According to Greek mythology, all the poisonous and venomous creatures of the desert came from the blood dripping from a severed head being carried by Perseus. Who's bloody head supposedly gave rise to these poisonous creatures?

Medusa, one of the Gorgon sisters.

○   The famous Roman historian and scientist, Pliny the Elder, was killed in 79 A.D., by a cloud of sulphurous gas which had been released by what famous explosion he was studying?

The eruption of Mount Vesuvius.

○   When food spoils there is always the possibility of food poisoning. But there is one food that does NOT spoil with time. What food has been removed in an edible state from ancient Egyptian tombs?

Honey.

○   In the year 82 B.C., the Roman world was first exposed to the *Lex Cornelia*. What was it?

The first law against poisoning.

○   Plutarch described an incident which occurred to the army lead by Mark Anthony against the Parthians, when soldiers consumed a forage plant causing an individual to lose *"all memory and would busy himself in turning over every stone he met with...till at last they were carried off by bilious vomiting...."* What toxic ingredient was felt to have caused this mass military casualty?

Aconite.

○ **In Roman legendary history, the sister of Hannibal died after drinking a bowl of poison sent to her by Masinissa, king of the Numidians. Her last words were:** *"If my husband has for his new wife no better gift than a cup of death, I bow to his will and accept what he bestows. I might have died more honorably if I had not wedded so near my funeral."* **What was her name?**

Sophonisba.

○ **Most people believe that the Egyptian Queen, Cleopatra, committed suicide with the bite of an asp. But, this could not have been true. Why?**

It is an *anachorism* (out of geographic placement), as "Asps" are not native to Egypt. She probably used an "Egyptian Cobra."

○ **The first reference to what potent marine toxin goes back some 4,500 years to the death, thought to be from it, of the Egyptian Pharaoh** *Ti*?

Tetrodotoxin.

○ **What famous conquering Carthaginian general ended his life by drinking poisoned wine, saying** *"It is time now to end the great anxiety of the Romans, who have grown weary waiting for the death of a hated old man"*?

Hannibal (249-183 B.C.).

○ **What observant Roman poet penned the lines:** *"Mixed with blood, the serpent's poison kills; the bite conveys it. Death lurks in the teeth. Swallowing it worked no harm"*?

Lucan.

○ **The rulers of what ancient kingdom incorporated in their regal headdress a vulture (***"Nehkbet"***) and a cobra (***"Wadjet"*** or** *"Uraeus"***)?**

Ancient Egypt.

○ **Who's death was described by the following:** *"When the fatal cup was brought, he asked what it was necessary for him to do. 'Nothing more', replied the servant of the judges, 'then as soon as you have drunk of the draught, to walk about until you find your legs become weary and afterwards lie down upon your bed.."*?

Socrates, as written by Plato in the *Phaedo*.

○ **Somewhere in the time period between 1,000 B.C. and 600 B.C., the Hindu physician Susrata, in a work titled the** *Arthara Vida***, first described in the medical literature what treatment for envenomation?**

The use of tourniquet, incision, and suction.

○   We all know that some of the insecticides can be toxic. But did you know that the ancient Chinese some 2,000 years ago, were thought to have used the first insecticide, for fleas. What was the plant insecticide they used?

Powdered chrysanthemums.

○   Living from 502-575 A.D., he was the first Christian physician of note, and his writings on poisons are among the best in antiquity. Who was he?

Aetios (Aetius) of Amida.

○   In the Roman writings of Ovid, what is referred to as the *"step-mother's poison"*?

"Wolfsbane."

○   She was known as *"The Mistress of Charms and Spells,"* the *"Terrible Goddess,"* the *"Controller of noxious poisons."* She is the earliest known deity associated with poisons. By what name did the Sumerians call her in 4,500 B.C.?

Gula.

○   This general was known as the *"Tyrant of Sicily."* He was born the son of a potter, and died in 289 B.C., when he was administered poison by his grandson. What was his name?

Agathocles.

○   This Athenian statesman who was regarded as one of the greatest Greek orators, took poison in 322 B.C., to escape his enemies. Who was he?

Demosthenes.

○   If you were having a conversation with an ancient Greek and he told you he was *"intoxicated,"* what would he actually mean?

He had been shot with a poisoned arrow - from the Greek word, *"toxicon"* signifying a bow (used to shoot poison-tipped arrows).

○   It has been called the *"Queen Mother of Poisons"* and has been noted by historians for over 2,000 years. It is also said to have been derived from the Greek word for javelin or arrow because some barbarous nations employed the juice to poison their arrows and spears. What is the common name for this poison?

Aconite.

○   This man, the son of Emperor Claudius, was set aside by Agrippina in favor of her son Nero. He was poisoned by Nero in 55 A.D. What was his name?

Britannicus.

O   The ancients widely believed in the physiological effects of *"bull's blood."* Did they think it was a poison or an antidote?

Poison.

O   This famous Greek mythical hero was driven to suicide by a transdermal poison made from the blood of a *Centaur*. The poison was administered to him by his wife, thinking it would act as a love potion. Who was this tragic husband?

Hercules.

O   This ancient writer (204-138 B.C.) wrote two treatises on poisons, one on snakes, and one on plants. Who was he?

Nicander of Colophon.

O   In 400 B.C., the troops of *"Cyrus the Younger,"* ate local honey near Trabzon in the northeastern Turkey. According to Xenophon, the troops were leveled *"in great numbers, as if there had been a defeat; and there was general dejection."* What is the postulated honey-borne cause of the army's problems?

The honey had come from the nectar of the *Rhododendron ponticum*, which contains toxic diterpenes called *"grayanotoxins."*

O   In what country was the first law against criminal poisoning passed, by Sulla, in 82 B.C.?

Rome, Italy. Penalty was confiscation of property and exile, or exposure to wild beasts.

O   It has been proposed that the great Roman Empire had a toxic decline. What is thought to have been the toxic cause?

Lead.

O   In India, what practice did the Brahmins put into place to discourage the domestic poisoning of husbands by their wives?

Suttee, or self-immolation of a wife on her husband's funeral pyre.

O   Among the famous antidotes of antiquity, was a peculiar clay which came from the Island of Lemnos. The red clay was excavated with great ceremony, from the side of a certain hill on the 6th of August. The Greeks then stamped or sealed the earth with a representation of the goddess *Diana*. It had a universal reputation as an antidote to all poisons, and drinking vessels were made from the material. By what name was this material known?

"Terra Sigillata."

○ In the 3rd Century A.D., the Emperor Hadrian, concocted a 40 ingredient antidote that was to rival the popular *"theriaca"* and *"mithridate"* of the period. What was it called?

"Adrianus."

○ In the Alexandrian and Roman period, what word meant both a poison or a medicine?

"Medicamentus."

○ A popular antidote of the ancients was an imprinted earth called *"Terra Mellitea,"* which came from the island of Malta. For what poisonous encounters was it especially used?

The bites of serpents.

○ During his Persian campaign the army of Alexander the Great lost horses which had fed on this shrub, and some soldiers died who had grilled meat on skewers made from this wood. What plant was the source of this calamity?

Nerium oleander.

○ In his treatise *Materia medica*, this physician in Nero's court, categorized poisons by their origin, as animal, vegetable, or mineral. What was this physician's name?

Dioscorides (40-80 A.D.).

○ List the four mineral poisons of antiquity?

Lead, Arsenic, Mercury, and Antimony.

○ According to Greek mythology, *Orion* was a great hunter, but when he dared to defy *Artemis*, she then produced what toxic encounter for *Orion*, that killed him?

A scorpion's sting.

○ In Ancient Egypt, this hawk-headed god was called the *"stopper of snakes,"* and people often carried his image as a charm against snakebite. What was his name?

Horus.

○ In Ancient Egypt, *"Selket,"* was the goddess of what venomous animal?

The scorpion.

○ In 201 B.C., Clisthenes contaminated a besieged city's drinking water with what plant to weaken thein habitants?

Hellebore.

❍   **In ancient India what activity was associated with individuals known as *"dhatureas"*?**

They used the seeds of the *Datura* to incapacitate their victims, so they could rob them.

❍   **When Boudicca, warrior Queen of the *Iceni*, was defeated in battle by the Roman forces under Seutonius Paulinus, in 61 A.D., she took poison rather than be captured alive. In what country did this event take place?**

Britain.

❍   **In the third century B.C., the Chinese Ch'in emperor *Shih Huang Ti*, who is notable for uniting China and constructing the Great Wall, is supposed to have died from ingesting elixir containing toxic compounds. Why was he testing these substances?**

He was seeking a source of immortality.

❍   **The use of the toxic agent *"fe she,"* was described in Chinese pharmacopoeias of the 8th Century A.D., and in *"The Great Pharmacopoeia"* of Shi-zen Li of the 16th Century. What was the source of this medicinal substance?**

The snake *Agkistrodon blomhofii brevicaudus*, "Chinese Mamushi."

❍   **Of the constellation that make up the twelve signs of the *Zodiac*, which one is based on a venomous creature?**

"Scorpio," the scorpion.

❍   **In 65 A.D., what Roman philosopher and statesman, having fallen out of favor with Emperor Nero, opened his veins and drank Hemlock, thus committing suicide?**

Seneca.

❍   **If your Roman host offered you the use of a *"pinna"* after dinner, for what purpose is it to be used?**

To induce vomiting by tickling the throat, it is a *"vomiting feather."*

❍   **The most prominent, as well as the most remorseless of the Greek poisoners, was the wife of Philip of Macedon, and mother of Alexander the Great. What was her name?**

Olympias.

❍   **Toffana was a notorious poisoner in Naples, Italy, and she sold her arsenical solutions to married women to do in their husbands. By what name was her bottle of poison usually labeled?**

"Manna of St. Nicholas of Bari."

O   **One of his most masterful orations was in defense of Cluentius who had been accused of poisoning. Who was this great orator?**

Cicero.

O   **One of the first documented cases of poisoning by Carbon monoxide, was in 364 A.D., and involved the death of what Roman emperor?**

Jovian.

O   **The death of what great Arabian physician was thought to be due to *"Mithridatic,"* which had an excess amount of opium?**

Avicenna (980-1037 A.D.).

O   **When the remains of the *"Iceman"* were discovered in the *Otzal Alps* in 1991, many of his personal effects were also recovered. His unfinished bow was found to be made of the wood of a toxic plant. What plant material was used?**

Yew, *Taxus baccata.*

O   **The book of *Arnald of Villanove*, written at the end of the 1200s, stated that an antidote against poison was served well by the picture of a man holding a dead object in his right hand and its tail in his left hand. What object was the person supposed to be holding?**

A dead serpent.

O   **It is said that the ancient Greeks knew of Arsenic and its toxic properties, in the form of *"Realgar."* By what chemical name is this substance better known?**

Arsenic disulfide.

O   **The *"Homeric Hymn to Hermes,"* from 8-6 B.C., describes *"melissae"* or *"bee-oracles"* who prophesied under the influences of honey. What component of the honey was thought to produce hypnotic effects?**

Grayanotoxins, from members of the Heath family of plants.

O   **In ancient Rome, what toxicological function was fulfilled by a *"pregustatore"*?**

Food tasting.

O   **What venomous animal was associated with the following ancient Egyptian deities: *"Mertseger," "Buto,"* and *"Renenet"*?**

The snake.

❍   **Norse mythology tells the story of the poisoning of what major hero by the great serpent *"Midgard"*?**

Thor.

❍   **In the 1970s, there occurred quite a stir in the world of Egyptology, when what two potentially toxic substances were discovered during the drug analysis of ancient mummy remains?**

Nicotine and cocaine.

❍   **On the island of *Ceros*, what plant was used by the ancients to poison people of no further value to the State?**

Aconite, *Aconitum napellus.*

❍   **In Greek legend, the son of Peleus was killed during the *Trojan War* when Paris fired a poisoned arrow that struck this warrior in the foot. Who was he?**

Achilles.

❍   **In southern Yugoslavian legend, it tells that *Wotan*, king of the gods, rides on his white horse, pursued by devils. The red and white flecks of foam that fall to the ground from his horse's mouth grow into the next year's crop of what mushroom?**

"Fly Agaric," *Amanita muscaria.*

❍   **According to the *Odyssey*, when Athena first met Odysseus, what toxic search was he carrying out?**

He was seeking the deadly poison [possibly Aconite] to anoint his bronze-tipped arrows.

❍   **Here are clues to the identity of a mythological character. FIRST CLUE: I was the greatest of mortal hunters in Greek mythology. SECOND CLUE: Artemis loved me, so Apollo sent a scorpion to sting me. THIRD CLUE: After my death, the Gods set my image in the sky where you can find my constellation by my belt and dagger.**

Orion.

❍   **List the plants which were considered the quartet of ancient poisons?**

(a) *Conium maculatum* "Poison Hemlock," (b) "Hellebore," (c) *Aconitum napellus* "Monkshood" or "Woolf's Bane," (d) *Atropa belladonna* "Deadly Nightshade."

❍   **In Greek mythology, it is said that *Orpheus* sang before *Hades*, asking for the release of the love of his life, *Eurydice*, who had died from what poisonous encounter?**

She died from the bite of a Viper.

○   **The writer Plutarch wrote of the last king of Pergamus:** *"And [he] used to grow poisonous plants, not only henbane and hellebore, but also hemlock, aconite, and dorycnium, sowing and planting them himself in the royal gardens, and making it his business to know their juices and fruits, and to collect these at the proper season."* **Who was the royal poison devotee?**

Attalus Philometor.

HISTORY: MILITARY

○ The *Treaty of Versailles* forced the Germans to relinquish their remedy for fever and rheumatism. What was this patented, but potentially toxic remedy?

Aspirin.

○ Its use was outlawed by the *Geneva Convention*. It was used by the Italians in Ethiopia in 1936, and by the Japanese at the battle of *Ichang*, China, on October 20, 1941. Winston Churchill had every intention of using it if the Germans invaded England in 1940. What was it?

Poison gas.

○ Near the closing days of World War II, there were many suicides in the Berlin bunker of Adolf Hitler, involving cyanide. Before the Potassium cyanide was used, it was first tested by Professor Werner Haase (substitute physician to Hitler). How did he test its deadly effectiveness?

The cyanide was tested effectively on Hitler's German shepherd dog, *"Blondi."*

○ In World War I, at least 1.3 million men were wounded by poisonous gas, and 91,000 of them died. What little known German Corporal, so wounded, later went on to become a prominent figure in post World War I Germany?

Adolf Hitler.

○ In the American Civil War, at the battle of Gettysburg, what General was supposedly so weakened by dysentery, that he agreed to the ill fated *"Pickett's Charge"*?

Robert E. Lee.

○ The worst chemical agent disaster in World War II, occurred on July 2, 1943, in the port of Bari, Italy, when a German Luftwaffe bomber blew up the Liberty ship *"SS John Harvey,"* which carried a secret cargo of 2,000 *M47A1* aerial bombs, containing 100 tons of a toxic chemical. The resultant contamination of the harbor area resulted in about 650 serous military cases and the death of over 1,000 Italian civilians within a few days. What was the toxic content of the cargo on this ship?

Distilled Mustard Gas, or *HD*, or Dichlorodiethylsulfide.

❍   The toxicological world is well informed of the dangers of dioxins in the herbicide *"Agent Orange,"* which was used in Viet Nam. But where did it get the colorful part of its name?

It was derived from the color of the bands painted around the center of the 55 gallon drums which contained the herbicide.

❍   When the German *"blitz"* began over England in *World War II*, what was done at the London Zoo to protect the general British population?

All the venomous snakes were killed, to prevent any accidental escape.

❍   The *"kamikaze"* was to Japanese military tactics, as what is to the *Hymenoptera*?

The Honeybee, a successful attack costs it its life.

❍   A great controversy exists concerning the intentional murdering of troops at the city of Jaffa, during the *Syrian Campaign* of 1799. It is alleged that the commanding general had his wounded troops euthanized by a pharmacist who administered Laudanum (Tincture of Opium) to an estimated 7 to 500 soldiers. What was the name of the French general who supposedly gave the orders?

Napoleon Bonaparte.

❍   Just after July 3, 1863, many of the trees around this small Pennsylvania town began dying from lead poisoning, due to the large number of leaded foreign bodies which had been embedded in the wood. What is the name of this town, which experienced this horrendous shooting event during the American Civil War?

Gettysburg, Pennsylvania.

❍   During the American Civil War (1861-1865), Northerners who sympathized with the southern cause, were given a nickname the same as a venomous creature. What was this nickname?

"Copperheads."

❍   Wounded during the siege of the Castle Biano in 1507, his final words being: *"I die unprepared."* So ended the life of one of the most notorious poisoners of the period. Who was he?

Cesare Borgia.

❍   On June 18, 1815, this military general was defeated in a now famous battle. His loss was complicated when his senses were probably dulled by opium he had been administered to relieve the pain of his swollen hemorrhoids. Who was this political power?

Napoleon Bonaparte, at Waterloo.

❍   **During World War II, the skull and crossbones could be found as an insignia on what German military group?**

SS, or *Schutzstaffel.*

❍   **What kind of venomous snake did the military name a helicopter after?**

"Cobra."

❍   **In 1941, during World War II, this priest, and to be Catholic Saint, was martyred at Auschwitz by lethal injection when he voluntarily exchanged himself for a Polish prisoner. Who was he?**

St. Maximilien Kolbe.

❍   **Born in 1833, Pauline Cushman, was a famous Northern female spy during the American Civil War. In 1893, she died from a suicidal overdose of what drug popular during the period?**

Opium.

❍   **During the Nepalese War of 1814-1816, Gurkhas extracted what plant poison which they called *"bikh,"* and used to poison water wells that would be used by British troops?**

Aconitum spicatum.

❍   **During the American Civil War, a form of bacterial warfare was carried out to contaminate ponds and lakes, thus forcing the opposing troops to carry large supplies of drinking water, that would slow down their advance. What was placed in these bodies of water to contaminate them?**

The bodies of dead animals (*i.e.* sheep and pigs).

❍   **In 1962, the United States Army, took out a patent to use what powdered toxic seeds as a potential agent in chemical warfare?**

Castor Bean, *Ricinus communis*

❍   **During World War I, at the Second Battle of Ypres, around the village of Langemark, Belgium, on April 22, 1915, the German forces marked the beginning of modern chemical warfare with the mass release of 6,000 cylinders of what toxic gas upon French and Canadian troops resulting in 20,000 casualties?**

Chlorine.

❍   **It is flown in daily from Yemen and Turkey, and it was of some concern to soldiers in 1992, who were assigned to the military operations in Somalia, where it is chewed by the residents for its stimulant effects. What is it?**

"Khat," *Catha edulis.*

O   **Developed in England in 1952, this chemical is the world's most powerful known nerve gas, with a *LD* of 100 *mg/min/m³* airborne or 0.3 *mg* orally. By what two letters is this nerve gas known?**

VX.

O   **In 1960, the spy pilot Francis Gary Powers was shot down over the Soviet Union in the famous *"U-2"* incident. He carried a hollow silver dollar containing a needle covered with a poisonous substance, to be used for suicidal purposes in case of capture. What poison was provided for that purpose?**

Saxitoxin, obtained from shellfish.

O   **What addicting drug did Britain and China fight a war over?**

"The Opium War" (1839-1842).

O   ***"Bullfight Brandy"* was a drink concocted by members of the famous *"Merrill's Marauders"* in Burma during World War II. The intoxicating beverage usually made the drinker almost uncontrollable. What was probably the major psychoactive ingredient that caused this effect?**

Marijuana.

O   **World War II was the first war in history where more soldiers died from their wounds than from disease. The wide use of what now banned insecticide is most likely credited with this historical change?**

DDT.

O   **In Bolivia, in 1983, what former Nazi, known as *"The Butcher of Lyon,"* was arrested for dealing in cocaine?**

Klaus Barbie.

O   **In 1720, troops of Czar Peter the Great, were defeated, not by the Turkish empire, but by what toxic substance growing in the *Volga Valley* which poisoned both man and beast?**

Ergot.

O   **This sect, founded in Persia in 1090, by Hassan ben Sabbah (the *"Old Man of the Mountains"*), was a band of military-religious fanatics. Their name was derived from *"hashish,"* an intoxicating drink which they are said to have used to prepare themselves for their orgies of massacre. What was the name of this group, which is still in popular use today?**

"Assassins."

❍   **This rapid acting poison was carried by some members of the *O.S.* during World War II, as a suicidal agent in case of capture. What is the name of this chemical terminating agent?**

Cyanide, or salts of cyanide.

❍   **By some estimates, more than 80% of all chemical agent fatalities in World War I, were from what chemical?**

"Phosgene," Carbonyl chloride, $COCl_2$.

❍   **At the Battle of North Taku Fort, during the China War of 1860, the British troops faced pots of what chemical substance thrown at them by the Chinese defenders?**

Caustic Soda (Sodium hydroxide).

❍   **During World War II, many English aviation ground crewman were killed or injured when they stepped on what substance which had been soaked by liquid oxygen spilled from refills of pilot's breathing apparatus?**

Asphalt.

❍   **During the American Civil War, there was a patent issued for a canon shell which was filled with a toxic chemical. Even though it was never used, what was proposed for use in this first, in American chemical warfare munition?**

Chlorine.

❍   **A toxic product named *Zyklon B* was used in large quantities during World War II. For what was it used?**

It was the source of Hydrogen cyanide that the Germans used in their extermination camps.

❍   **Being falsely implicated in an attempt on the life of Hitler, this famous German military commander was forced to commit suicide, in 1944, by taking poison. Who was he?**

Field Marshall Erwin Eugene Rommel.

❍   **During the 1991 Persian Gulf War, the world became very conscious of the potential for chemical warfare. Give the common names of the four major nerve gas agents.**

Taubin (or *GA*), Sarin (or *GB*), Soman (or *GD*), and *VX*.

❍   **World War II saw the widespread use of legally authorized drugs among the troops. German Panzer troops used this drug to eliminate fatigue and maintain** physical endurance, and some historians have even linked many of the German atrocities to the abuse of what drug substance?

Amphetamines.

❍   In 1862, John Doughty suggested to the Union's Secretary of War that special artillery shells be filled with what toxic compound to use against the Confederate forces?

Chlorine.

❍   During World War II, *"POISON"* was the military code name for what ocean body of water?

The Indian Ocean.

❍   In Viet Nam, the U.S. *4th Infantry Division*, was also known by what toxic nick name?

The *"Poison Ivy"* Division.

❍   It was a combination of *2,4-D*, *2,4,5-T*, with small amounts of *TCDD*, and it caused many claims involved with military service. What is the more common name of this mixture?

"Agent Orange."

❍   From 1935-1945, the infamous *"Unit 731"* was secretly operated by the Japanese, to conduct experiments in germ and chemical warfare. In what country did this top-secret operation take the lives of over 3,000 prisoners?

Harbin, China.

❍   During the Normandy Invasion of World War II, the code name for the plan to break out from the area of *St. Lo*, France, was the same as a venomous animal. What was the code name?

"Operation Cobra."

❍   During World War II, the nickname for the short German General Gotthard Heinrici used by his friends and enemies was *"Unser Giftwerg"*? What did it mean?

"Our poison dwarf."

❍   The American *"P-61"* night fighter was the largest and most powerful aircraft in World War II, and was named for a toxic critter. For what animal was it named?

"Black Widow."

O   During World War II, a Britisher named E. Clifton James, served in the role as a double for Field Marshall, Bernard Montgomery, in order to fool the Germans on the true target of the *D-Day* invasion. This operation was given a code name, the same as a venomous snake. What was it?

"Operation Copperhead."

O   A special tank was used by the British in North Africa during World War II, which had a flail on the front in order to detonate mines. It was named after a toxic critter. What was the name?

"Scorpion."

O   It is well known that during the Viet Nam war, there was a defoliating agent used called *"Agent Orange,"* but there were also two other herbicides used with similar colorful names. What were the two colors?

"Agent Purple," and *"Agent White."*

O   The Carthaginians are reported to have defeated a Roman expeditionary force in the third century B.C., by catapulting pots containing what toxic agent into their ships?

Live snakes.

O   Probably the greatest number of snake bites suffered by the armed forces of the United States occurred during World War II, during their military campaign on what Pacific island?

Okinawa. Mostly from the *"Habu."*

O   During World War I, in an attempt to conserve food, the British government recommended that people eat what plant leaf that proved to have toxic consequences?

Rhubarb.

O   During the 11th Century, what emperor conquered an Italian town by contaminating its water supply with the carcasses of dead animals?

Emperor Frederick Barbarossa.

O   During the 1960s, the *CIA* concocted a plan to use poison to assassinate what political leader of the African Congo?

Patrice Lumumba.

O   What 1925 protocol banned the use of poisons in warfare?

The Geneva Protocol.

❍   The French included this poison among *"les grands toxiques,"* and Napoleon III used it as a war gas as early as 1865. What was this chemical agent?

Hydrogen cyanide.

❍   Each member of the flight crew that climbed on board their plane carried Cyanide in case they were captured by the enemy. What was the target, in 1945, of the *"Enola Gay"*?

Hiroshima, Japan – dropping of the first atomic bomb.

❍   During the Crimean War, at the siege of Sebastopol in 1855, Admiral Lord Dundonald, submitted a plan to use what toxic fumes on the Russian forts?

Sulphur.

❍   During World War II, what were *"L pills"*?

The designation for Potassium cyanide pills carried by Allied agents in occupied countries.

❍   Dying from the consequences of food poisoning in Mobile, Alabama on August 30, 1877, Raphael Semmes, had been captain of a Confederate ship which was probably one of the most successful sea raiders in military history. What was the name of this feared Confederate military vessel?

CSS *"Alabama,"* sunk off Cherbourg, France, June 19, 1864.

❍   In 1899, during the Boer War, the British filled some of their artillery shells with what toxic chemical in order to try to induce vomiting in the enemy troops?

Picric acid.

❍   Against what ethnic group did Iraq's Saddam Hussein use poison gas?

The *Kurds.*

❍   Embalmers during the American Civil War injected what toxic compound into dead soldiers to temporarily preserve them for shipment to their home towns for burial?

Mercuric chloride.

❍   During World War I, this chemical was used as a war gas. It was called *"D-Stoff,"* or *"Rationite."* What chemical was so used?

Dimethyl sulphate.

❍   During World War II, what chemical substance was included in a soldier's *"survival pack"* to assist his stamina and decrease his need for food?

Amphetamine.

❍   **In World War I, over 80% of poison gas fatalities resulted from what gas?**

Phosgene, Carbonyl chloride.

❍   **In 1722, at the Battle of Astrakahn, the Russian cavalry was defeated by the Turks because of what poisonous affliction that had affected some of the Russian troops?**

Ergotism.

❍   **During the "Battle of Britain," much fame was gained by the British fighter plane known as the *"Spitfire,"* yet the designer of the plane preferred to name it after a quick moving venomous mammal. What name did he prefer?**

The *"Shrew."*

❍   **According to the July 1968 issue of *Civil War Times*, there was a Confederate proposal to deliver poison gas onto Union troops by what unique method?**

They planned to drop it from manned balloons.

❍   **What was the first documented use of nerve agents on a battlefield?**

In 1988, Iraq used Sarin against the Kurds.

❍   **It has been stated that British *MI-6* planned to use a biological weapon in the assassination of Nazi leader Reinhard Heydrich. What substance did they plan to use?**

Botulinus toxin.

❍   **During World War II, the German scientists tested poison bullets for use in combat. With what toxic plant substance did they experiment?**

Aconitine.

❍   **Questions have arisen concerning veterans of the "Persian Gulf War," that may be related to chemical or drug exposures. One of the substances questioned is the drug given to the troops in "blister packs" to take in case of exposure to the nerve gas Sarin. Answer the following about this antidote: (a) What was the name of this protective drug, (b) In what disease state is this drug normally used, (c) Does this drug cross the blood-brain barrier?**

(a) Pyridostigmine bromide, "Mestinon," (b) Myasthenia gravis, (c) No, because of its ionic character.

❍   **During the Persian Gulf War, what term, borrowed from the film *Ghostbusters*, did soldiers use to describe being hit by a chemical weapon?**

"Slimed."

O   **During World War II, the Japanese had a plan to create an Israel-like homeland in Asia for Jews, which would be under Japanese control, thus giving them leverage and international support. This plan was named for a very toxic marine creature. What was the name?**

The *"Fugu Plan."*

O   **In 1998, there was a dispute between the media and the military that during September 1970, U.S. military forces supposedly used Sarin (*GB*) nerve gas during a raid into Laos in order to eliminate American defectors. What was the name of this military mission?**

"Operation Tailwind."

O   **In 1944, an operation by *British Special Operations Executive (SOE)* to subvert ex-Soviet soldiers in German service in Germany and the occupied European nations was named after a deadly snake. What snake's name was the code name?**

"Operation *Mamba*."

O   **What poisonous chemical warfare agent was commonly called the "*King of the Battle Gases*"?**

"Mustard Gas," or Sulphur mustard.

O   **The first casualty of the American Civil War was not by bullet or bayonet, but by venom. In this incident, (a) What creature caused the casualty? (b) In what State is this offending creature on display?**

(a) Eastern Coral Snake, (b) Augusta, Georgia.

O   **During World War II, a gas mask for children was designed with the face of a popular cartoon character. What character was used?**

Mickey Mouse.

O   **In 1675, in the city of Strasbourg, the French and Germans signed a treaty to ban the use of what type of poisoned military weapon?**

Poisoned bullets.

O   **On October 27, 1914, the Germans exposed the British forces to the chemical Dianisidine chlorosulfate. By what means was the chemical delivered?**

The firing of 3,000 artillery shells (sized 105 *mm*).

O   **When we have a cold today, we commonly grab a Kleenex®, but for what toxicological use were they originally developed?**

They were originally manufactured for use as gas mask filters in World War I.

❍   **On the big island of Hawaii, in 1790, *Keoua* sent a group of warriors to do battle with the forces of *King Kamehameha*. However the attacking forces were annihilated when they were killed by toxic forces. What natural force killed them?**

The *Kilauea* volcano erupted and poured out toxic gases.

❍   **During the Franco-Prussian war, Napoleon III, proposed that the bayonets of the French troops be dipped into what toxic compound?**

Cyanide.

❍   **The term *"tear gas"* is really a misnomer. What is technically wrong with the term?**

It is actually an aerosolized solid.

❍   **In World War I, the French used approximately 4,000 tons of a substance called *"vincennite."* What was the toxic chemical in this substance?**

Cyanide.

❍   **Identify the following chemical warfare agents, by their characteristic odor: (a) geraniums, (b) almonds, (c) garlic or onion, (d) new mown hay or freshly cut grass or corn, (e) rotting fruit.**

Lewesite [*L*], (b) Hydrogen cyanide [*AC*], (c) Mustard [*HD*], (d) phosgene [*CG*], (e) Ethyldichloroarsine [*ED*].

HISTORY: MODERN

❍   In 1916, in Russia, there was an assassination attempt on the life of a religious leader who was very influential with the *Tsarina*. Although he was fed massive doses of cyanide in chocolate cake by Dr. Lasovert and Prince Yussupov, he did not die. He was next shot multiple times, but his death was ultimately due to being drowned in the *Neva River*. What was the name of this sturdy victim?

Grigori Yefimovich Rasputin (1871-1916).

❍   *Wall Street* is associated with high financial trading, and *Hollywood* and *Vine* is associated with movie stars. What district in San Francisco, California was associated with flower children and the drug culture in the 1960s?

Haight and Ashbury.

❍   In what Century did Louis *XIV* require all French apothecaries to first maintain a *"poison register,"* which would require that purchasers sign and declare the purpose for which the poison was being purchased?

The 17th Century, actually in the year 1662.

❍   In 1809, Nicholas Appert, a Parisian candy maker, was awarded a 12,000 franc prize by Napoleon Bonaparte, for originating what process against intoxications, that allowed the General to better prepare for his campaign into Russia?

Food preservation by canning.

❍   In 1604, James I of England, wrote the following about a certain commonly used toxic substance: *"A custome lothsome to the eye, hateful to the nose, harmfull to the braine, dangerous to the lungs, and the blacke stinking fume thereof, neerest resembling the horrible Stygian smoke of the pit that is bottomless."* About what substance was he writing?

Tobacco, in his *Counterblaste to Tobacco.*

❍   What was the relationship of Pope Alexander *VI* and the infamous poisoner Rodrigo Borgia (1431?-1503), father of Cesare and Lucretia Borgia?

They were one in the same person!

❍   In 1980, when French police and intelligence personnel raided a "safe house" at *41A Chaillot St.*, Paris, they were surprised to find what toxic agent being manufactured, by the German *"Red Army Faction"* for potential terrorist use?

Botulinus toxin.

❍ **In 1936, King George *V* of England supposedly died peacefully after a long illness. However, the notes of Lord Dawson, the King's personal physician, published in 1986, revealed that the doctor had carried out euthanasia on the King by administering an injection of what two toxic substances?**

Morphine and cocaine.

❍ **Poisons are often associated with witches. After the mass hysteria which lead to the *"Witch Trials"* of 1692 in Salem, Massachusetts, how many of the condemned 20 women were burned at the stake?**

None! 19 were hanged, and one pressed to death.

❍ **In France, in the 1670s, what was the *"Affair of Poisons"*?**

When some women who claimed to have supernatural powers sold poisons for their customers to dispose of unwanted spouses.

❍ **About the year 1035 A.D., the Scots under *Duncan I* destroyed the Scandinavian army under King Sven Canute, by adding what poisonous solanaceous plant to meal which they used to prepare their food?**

Atropa belladonna, or "Deadly Nightshade."

❍ **At the time of the French Revolution in 1798, what was the most popular suicidal poison?**

Mercuric chloride, $HgCl_2$.

❍ **In 1989, the historian Mary Kilburne Mattossian put forth the theory that an event in France in the spring of 1789, which is known as the *"Great Fear"* was NOT caused by the French Revolution, but actually by food contaminated with what toxic agent?**

Ergot fungus.

❍ **Name the four toxic ingredients of *"witches' ointment"* or *"flying mixtures"* that was supposedly used by "witches" to anoint themselves in preparation for the "witches' Sabbath," as recorded by Johannes Wierius in 1566?**

Mandrake, belladonna, henbane, and stramonium.

❍ **In the 13th century, Peter of Abanos, in his work *De Venenis*, divided all poisons into what three major categories?**

Animal, vegetable, and mineral.

❍   Catherine de'Medici was such a notorious poisoner that when she married into the royal family of France, her uncle, Pope Clement *VII*, gave a gift to the French king to lessen the fear that she might practice her art on her husband's relatives. What was the gift?

A *"unicorn's horn."*

❍   In 1846, a British expedition led by Sir John Franklin, met disaster which led to the deaths of over 128 men. It is now theorized that the members of the expedition suffered from lead poisoning which resulted in emaciation and mental problems leading up to their desperate and disastrous trek toward rescue. Answer the following about this event: (a) What is theorized to have been the source of lead which intoxicated the crew, (b) What route was this unfortunate expedition attempting to explore?

(a) The solder from the seams of the tins used for foods, (b) The *"Northwest Passage."*

❍   In the history of the early Christian Church, one of Christ's apostles was challenged by Aristodemos, priest of Diana, to drink a cup of poison. This apostle is said to have made the sign of the cross on the cup, Satan flew from it like a dragon, and he then drank the now harmless liquid. Answer the following: (a) What is the name of this apostle, (b) What is the badge, or symbol, used by the Church for this apostle, which commemorates this event?

(a) John, (b) A cup with a winged serpent flying out of it.

❍   Which country was the first to have an epidemic of amphetamine abuse after World War II?

Japan.

❍   On April 18, 1864, Union and Confederate forces were engaged in the State of Arkansas, at a place with a toxic sounding name. Name the location?

"Poison Springs."

❍   In 1782, the Swedish chemist Carl Scheele is credited with the discovery of what toxic compound that, in 1786, resulted in his sudden death from it in a laboratory accident?

Hydrogen cyanide, HCN.

❍   The arrow poison of the Pygmies of Central Africa, an ingredient of which was red ants of which a single arrow was supposedly capable of killing an elephant, was described by what American explorer, who was in search of a famous British personage?

Henry Morton Stanley (1841-1904) searched for Dr. David Livingstone.

❍   **During the 1960s, it was held by the drug culture that one could get high from smoking the peel of what popular fruit, even though there was no known pharmacological basis for the effect?**

Bananas.

❍   **Due to an outbreak of criminal poisoning in 1480, this British monarch is said to have issued a law to the effect that** *"All persons are forbidden to bring home poison from which any Christian man or woman can take harm."* **What was the name of this king?**

Scotland's James *I*.

❍   **Emperor Leo *VI* of Byzantium (886-911 A.D.) produced an edict which forbade the eating of what food, due to it's potential harm to the people's health?**

Blood sausage, a notable source of botulism.

❍   **During the *"Dark Ages"* (476-1492 A.D.) the treatment of ailments including poisoning revolved around the theory of *"similis similibus."* What was the principle of this theory?**

Treating like with like.

❍   **What European emperor adopted the symbol of the bee as his royal symbol?**

Napoleon I (1769-1821).

❍   **The *Efik* tribe along the Niger River of Africa, became famous for their secret societies, which were responsible for keeping order among their neighbors. One of their most powerful weapons was trial by poison, in which an individual had to drink a potion made from what toxic substance?**

The seeds of the "Calabar" bean, *Physostigma venenosum*.

❍   **One of the earliest American flags of the late 1700s showed a rattlesnake on an open field. What warning motto appeared beneath the symbol?**

"Don't Tread On Me."

❍   **England's King Henry *VIII*, killed two of his six wives, but stood in constant fear of being poisoned by one in particular. Of which wife was he referring to when he said, *"We must thank God for having escaped from the hands of that venomous harlot"*?**

Anne Boleyn.

MISCELLANEOUS

O   In what year was the *American Association of Poison Control Centers* officially founded?

1958.

O   In order for an acetaminophen level to be most meaningful, it should be drawn NOT earlier than how many hours post exposure?

4 hours.

O   If the *DOT* were talking to the *NRC*, who would be talking to whom?

The *Department of Transportation* would be talking to the *Nuclear Regulatory Commission*.

O   This is a mathematical question. A child weighing 10 kg, ingests 20 ml of a 100 proof alcoholic beverage. How many *ml/kg* of pure ethanol did this patient ingest?

1 *ml/kg*.

O   In the following statement there is an inaccuracy. Indicate what is wrong with the following: *"Swinging through the jungle, Tarzan's yell startled the animal inhabitants. Sunning itself in the branches of a tree, a "Green Mamba" slithered away disturbed by the loud sound."*

Snakes can NOT hear airborne sounds, since they have no ear openings.

O   In the United States, its called the *"Right-to-Know" (RTK)* law, or the *"Hazard Communications Standard" (HCS)*, but what is the counterpart to this important legislation called in Canada?

"Workplace Hazardous Materials Information System" (WHMIS).

O   If you saw a *Sistrurus catenatus*, would you be most apt to eat it, run from it, or put it in a vase?

Run from it. It is the *"Massasauga"* rattlesnake.

O   On December 13, 1990, 12 members of a religious sect were found dead in Tijuana, Mexico, after a ceremony in which they were attempting to speak with the spirits of the dead. What poisonous substance was found to be involved in their deaths?

Carbon monoxide.

❍   **The *pH* at which a substance exists 50% ionized and 50% in a nonionized form, is called what?**

PKa.

❍   **As a rule of thumb, for compounds eliminated by *"first-order kinetics,"* after how many half-lives, should no significant amount of drug remain?**

5 to 6.

❍   **How many *milligrams* of the antidote Deferoxamine are required to bind 17 *milligrams* of elemental iron?**

200 *milligrams.*

❍   **What toxicological association was formed in 1964 in Tours, France?**

The *European Association of Poison Control Centers (EAPCC).*

❍   **In order for a salicylate level to be most meaningful, by showing peak concentrations, it should be drawn NOT less than how many hours post exposure?**

6 hours.

❍   **If one was playing the game *Scrabble*® , and spelled the word *"POISON,"* with no bonus-letter scores, how many points would one receive?**

8 points (P=3, O=1, I=1, S=1, O=1, N=1).

❍   **On October 21, 1958, the first meeting of individuals interested in poisons and their treatment, took place. What organizational name was given to this group?**

The *American Association of Poison Control Centers (AAPCC).*

❍   **What important measurement is obtained, when one divides the dose of a drug in milligrams, by the plasma drug concentration in milligrams per liter?**

The "volume of distribution" = *Vd* (in liters).

❍   **Under the law, why is homicidal poisoning almost always considered murder and never manslaughter?**

Because of premeditation, deliberation, and intent to kill.

❍   **The *FDA* uses five letters to stand for the different pregnancy categories, as they relate to drugs. What are the five letters which are used?**

A, B, C, D, and *X.*

○   *Clostridium botulinum* is NOT likely to grow and produce its toxin below what *pH* threshold?

pH 4.6.

○   What term was humorously defined in the *Journal of Irreproducible Results* as coming from the Greek for "I never liked dogs," and meaning: *"Animal testing based on the premise that if something makes a dog sick, it isn't good for humans. (Ignoring the obvious corollary that humans should therefore thrive by drinking from rain puddles and eating dead possum at the roadside").*

"Toxicology."

○   The *"Ames Test"* is a rapid *in vitro* test for the potential of a substance to be a mutagen. What living organism is the basis for the test?

The bacteria *Salmonella typhimurium* that lacks the enzyme necessary for histidine synthesis.

○   Founded in 1980, this group supports the option of active voluntary euthanasia for the terminally ill, quite often recommending the use of poisons or drugs. What is the name of this rather unique Society?

The National Hemlock Society.

○   Using the currently used modern radio communication phonetic alphabet (i.e. *"Alpha," "Bravo," "Charlie,"* etc.), how would you communicate the word *"POISON"*?

Papa - Oscar - India - Sierra - Oscar – November.

○   Emesis induced with Syrup of Ipecac, within one hour of ingestion, will remove approximately what percent of the ingested material?

30-40% (anywhere in this range is correct).

○   The labels of premixed fertilizers customarily bear a series of three numbers, for example *8-6-4*. What, in order, do these numbers stand for?

The % by weight of Nitrogen, Phosphorus, and Potassium.

○   If one takes morphine and mixes it with acetic anhydride, to acetylate the parent molecule, does it increase or decrease its addiction potential?

Increases. It produces Diacetylmorphine, also known as *"Heroin."*

○   Which solution contains more formaldehyde: an aqueous solution of 37% *w/v* formaldehyde, or a 100% *Formalin* solution?

Neither! They both contain the same amount of formaldehyde.

◯   In treating an overdose of Acetaminophen, an antidote called *NAC* is commonly used. In order to be most effective, this antidote should be given before how many hours post exposure have passed?

12 hours.

◯   In 1991, the *CDC* lowered its *"threshold of concern"* for lead in children's whole blood to how many micrograms per deciliter?

10 *mcg/dL*.

◯   In a popular fantasy role playing game called *"Advanced Dungeons and Dragons,"* a player's characters are sometimes allowed to use poisons on the characters of another player. But, according to the official rule book which is the only class of characters which can never use poisons?

The *Paladins*.

◯   In the United States, during execution by lethal injection, how many toxic chemicals enter the bloodstream of the condemned?

Three.

◯   In iron toxicology there is the memory aid *FSG359*. What does it mean?

It is used, as a memory aid, to help calculate the amount of elemental iron in the common salts: fumarate, sulfate, and gluconate.

◯   The state of New Jersey recently made it illegal for restaurants to serve eggs soft-boiled or sunny-side-up. What form of food poisoning is this law intended to prevent?

Salmonellosis.

◯   Cyanide has the odor of almonds. Approximately what % of the general population can detect this odor, the rest being *"odor blind"*?

40-60% (anywhere in this range is correct).

◯   Over the years there have been many symbols used on stickers and poison center educational literature. Identify the name of the following symbols from their descriptions: (a) A policeman with his hands crossed over his mouth, (b) A green faced man with a long purple tongue sticking out, (c) A green snake on an orange background, (d) A bright-green face with a tongue sticking out, (e) A fireman with red and yellow colors?

(a) *"Officer Ugg®,"* (b) *"Uncle Icky®,"* (c) *"SIOP®,"* (d) *"Mr. Yuk®,"* (e) *"Fireman Red®,"* developed by the U.S. military.

○   **What governmental agency or group would be responsible for investigating the following areas: (a) Hazardous chemicals while in transit? (b) Toxic waste materials? (c) Flammable fabrics? (d) Dairy products? (e) Food additives? (f) Chemicals in the workplace?**

(a) *DOT* or Department of Transportation, (b) *EPA* or Environmental Protection Agency, (c) *CPSC* or Consumer Product Safety Commission, (d) *USDA* or Department of Agriculture, (e) *FDA* or Food and Drug Administration, (f) *OSHA* or Occupational Safety and Health Administration.

○   **The old logo of the *American Academy of Clinical Toxicology (AACT)* had three different components in the design. What were the three different representations?**

Benzene ring, Coral snake, and Opium poppy.

○   **If you take the number of letters in the word *"antivenin,"* ADD the number of *FDA* approved snake antivenins in the United States, and DIVIDE by the number of shells found on the toxic marine animal known as *Conus textilis*, what number is generated?**

12 = (9 + 3)/1.

○   **If you take the number of letters in the word *"antidote,"* ADD the number of species of venomous lizards found in the United States, and MULTIPLY the result by the number of legs found on a *Bungarus fasciatus*, what number is generated?**

0 = (8 letters + 1 species "Gila Monster") x 0 legs on the snake known as the "Banded Krait."

○   **If all the alphabet were assigned numerical values from 1 for *A*, to 26 for *Z*, what would be the value of the word *POISON*?**

88 = (16 + 15 + 9 + 19 + 15 + 14).

○   **According to the *Poison Prevention Packaging Act Standard* of April 1974: (a) What % of children under five years of age must be unable to get into a child-resistant container (*CRC*), (b) What % of adults must have easy access to the CRC container, (c) What agency is responsible for administering the *Poison Prevention Packaging Act*?**

(a) 80%, (b) 90%, (c) The *Consumer Products Safety Commission (CPSC)*.

○   **You are called by a law enforcement officer at the scene of a tanker spill, who describes the numbers on an *NFPA* placard on the vehicle. What do each of the color categories red, blue, and yellow, represent?**

Red = Flammability, *Blue* = Health hazard, *Yellow* = Reactivity.

○   **If you take the number of letters in the word *"toxicology,"* ADD the number of legs found on a *Latrodectus mactans*, and DIVIDE by the number of known species of clinically significant venomous starfish, what number is generated?**

18 = (10 letters + 8 spider legs/1 *"Crown of Thorns"*).

○   **If you take the number of letters in the word *"poisons,"* ADD the number of legs found on a *Phidipus audax*, and then DIVIDE by the number of *FDA* approved antivenins for snakebite in the United States, what number is generated?**

5 = (7 letters + 8 legs on a *"Jumping Spider"*/3 antivenins).

○   *National Poison Prevention Week* **is celebrated each year in the United States, but how much do you know of its origin? Answer the following about this annual event: (a) What was the name of the Cape Giarardeau, Missouri, pharmacist who was the originator, prime mover behind, and could be called the *"Father"* of this Week, (b) In what year did the U.S. Congress pass the bill calling for an annual National Poison Prevention Week, (c) On what day of what month does** *National Poison Prevention Week* **begin each year?**

(a) Homer A. George, (b) 1961, (c) The third Sunday of March.

○   **In what year, and in what city, did the first pilot poison center begin operations in the United States?**

1953, Chicago, Illinois.

○   **What is the meaning of these quantity prefixes: (a) *nano-*, (b) *kilo-*, (c) *pico-*, (d) *deci-*, (e) *micro-*?**

(a) billionth, (b) thousand, (c) trillionth, (d) tenth, (e) millionth.

○   **One might think that *"3030"* and *"357 Magnum"* are only measurements for the calibers of ammunition. But what potentially toxic compounds also carry these names?**

Street drug stimulants containing caffeine and/or ephedrine.

○   **The ratio of a drug's toxic dose to its therapeutic dose, is referred to by what term?**

Therapeutic index.

○   **In toxicology the dose of poison that is required to cause death in one-half of the study population, is referred to as what?**

The LD_{50}.

❍   In 1954, the *Bulletin of the World Health Organization* published an article by Swaroop and Grab, which presented one of the first international epidemiological studies on the world mortality from encounters with what toxic agent?

Snakebite.

❍   Most toxicologists consider the *"universal antidote"* to be universally worthless, yet it could be purchased commercially under what registered trade name?

Unidote ®, or *Res-Q* ® .

❍   In the religious art of the 14th-16th centuries, what toxic animal was often used as an emblem of the Jewish people to symbolize perfidy?

The scorpion.

❍   In 1992, the United States aimed to block the import of a vodka which was distilled in Belgium, and test marketed in selected American cities, due to misleading advertising. What was the rather toxic sounding name of this product?

"Black Death."

❍   In the 1992 *"Solar and Electric 500 Race,"* there was a toxic emission from one of the electric-car vehicles, when an overheated battery released what toxic fumes?

Bromine.

❍   In the Christian religion, what symbol associated with toxicology represents *Golgotha,* or thoughts of life after death?

A skull with crossed bones at its base.

❍   In 1994, the blood alcohol limit for motorists in the United States was 100 *mg/dL*, but in Sweden, was the limit: 20, 100, or 200 *mg/dL*?

20 *mg/dL.*

❍   In 1992, the *L. A. Gear* company began production of high-tech sneakers with colored lights that flashed when the heels hit the ground. Some states considered these shoes a pollution hazard when disposed because of what toxic material in the lighting mechanism?

Mercury.

❍   What automobile line uses the same name as a toxic heavy metal?

Mercury.

❍   Both *Alfa Romeo* and *Fiat* made cars with the same name as what venomous creature?

"Spider."

❍   *Dodge* produced an automobile with the same name as what type of venomous snake?

"Viper."

❍   What car manufacturer produced a car known as the *"Stingray"*?

Chevrolet.

❍   In 1980, a group of extortionists demanded diamonds in exchange for information on food items they had poisoned with cyanide, in San Diego, California, and Colorado Springs, Colorado. What self-assumed name did they use for their group?

"Poison Gang."

❍   In 1995, some commonly used children's objects were changed from scents such as coconut, licorice, chocolate, blueberry, and bubblegum, to odors thought to be less inviting to children. What type of objects were these?

Crayons®.

❍   *"Poison"* along with *"Potsies,"* *"Chassies,"* *"Black Snake"* and *"Old Boiler,"* are game variations played with what objects?

Marbles.

❍   The following statement contains an inaccuracy. State what is the error. Collecting shellfish along the coast off *Rio de Janero*, your guide says that it is not safe to eat shellfish in months that do NOT contain the letter *"r."*

This rule of thumb only applies to locations in the Northern Hemisphere!

❍   In the embalming processes in America, why were metallic substances eventually banned?

Because the use of Hg, As, Pb and Zn, would cover up cases of homicidal poisoning.

❍   What custom used at culinary festivities today is thought to have it roots in a polite mannerism to assure one's companion that no poison had been mixed in his cup?

The practice of toasting and clinking of glasses.

❍   Landscape *Feng Shui*, for rationalizing good and bad land sites, has been practiced in China since the *Tang* dynasty. In this school of thought, bad energy lines are caused by the presence of sharp pointed objects or structures that are aimed at habitats. These objects are referred to by a term that has a warlike toxicological association. What are they called?

"poison arrows."

O   Most people are familiar with the near disaster of the *Apollo 13* flight to the moon. But there was a toxicological concern in the back of engineers' minds, if the space craft disintegrated upon return to earth. On board was 8.3 pounds of what very toxic chemical that would have been a disaster if released in the earth's atmosphere?

Plutonium, in the *SNAP-27* equipment used to supply energy for experiments on the lunar surface.

O   Toxicity has sometimes occurred in Asian populations from such toxic metals as Copper, Arsenic, Mercury, Lead, and Antimony used in a type of medicine, or philosophy of health, which originated about 2,000 B.C. The name of this type of medicine comes from the Hindi for *"the science of life."* By what name is this form of medicine better known?

Ayurvedic medicine.

O   Many men have met their destruction by ingestion of *Cinnabar* (Mercuric sulphide), and many more have fallen under the spell of the smell of the perfume *"Cinnabar."* By what company is this product made?

Estee Lauder.

O   A prison correctional torture in the early 1900s consisted of placing the inmate in a cell the walls of which were lined with slaked lime and then spraying the walls with water, and forcing the condemned to inhale the resulting caustic fumes for long periods of time, until their respiratory tract was raw. What was this process called?

The *"lime cell."*

O   In 1905, what popular store catalogue offered for 69 cents, a bottled antidote for those addicted to opium or morphine?

Sears Roebuck.

O   In order to diminish alcohol intoxication, in 1920, the U.S. banned its manufacture and sale by a Constitutional amendment. What is the number of this amendment?

18th.

O   In September 1997, the United States Federal government began a fifty million dollar, five year project, called the *"EGP"* to check human toxin vulnerability. What does the acronym *"EGP"* stand for?

"Environmental Genome Project."

❍ **According to 1998 economics, which toxic method of execution is cheaper to administer, lethal gas or lethal injection?**

Lethal injection, $346.51 *vs.* $371.03.

❍ **List the four major properties of a good antidote.**

(a) Either reverses or neutralizes the effect of the poison, (b) Has no reaction of its own, (c) Easy to administer, (d) Has no unpleasant side effects.

❍ **If one takes the numbers of letters in the words *"TOXIC DOSE,"* adds the number of known species of green-spored mushrooms in North America, and then multiplies by the number of different components in the old lay-public recipe for *"Universal Antidote,"* what number is generated?**

30 = (9 letters + 1 species (*Chlorophyllum molybdites*), x 3 components: tea, toast, and Milk of Magnesia.

❍ **Although the couple were murdered by the blows from an axe, it is also interesting to note that Cyanide was also found in their sugar bowl. What famous 1892 case, from Fall River, Massachusetts was the cause of this town scandal?**

The Lizzie Borden Case.

❍ **For many, Rochester, New York is considered the birthplace of clinical toxicology in the United States, with the production of a valuable reference work in the 1950s. Give the four last names of the authors of this work, and the title of the book.**

(a) Gleason, Gosselin, Hodge, and Smith, (b) *The Clinical Toxicology of Commercial Products.*

❍ **According to the doctrines of Tibetan Buddhism, there are five *"poisons"* (actually vices) that drive the life cycle. What are these five frailties?**

(a) Ignorance (or delusion), (b) Lust, (c) Hatred, (d) Pride, (e) Envy.

❍ **In 1997, Quaker Oats and the *Massachusetts Institute of Technology* agreed to pay $1.85 million to settle a law suite regarding an incident dating back to the 1940s and 1950s. What did they do that resulted in this suit?**

Boys at the Fernald School, Waltham, Mass., were given radioactive *Quaker Oats*® in an attempt to prove nutrients traveled throughout the body.

❍ **In 1998, the *U.S. Consumer Product Safety Commission*, recalled 3,700 backpacks with images of Disney's *"Mulan,"* because of what toxic problem?**

The artwork contained paint with high levels of lead.

○   **In 1998, 68 year old Nell Rein, a nursing home resident in Jackson, Mississippi, died in her bed from what unusual toxic encounter?**

She was swarmed by Fire Ants, while laying in bed.

○   **In the 1990s, the *"Beanie Baby"* craze was upon adults as well as children. Interestingly enough, six of the created characters were unquestionably based on animals with a known venomous nature. What type of creature was so depicted and what was the character's name?**

(a) *"Stinger"* the scorpion, (b) *"Bumble"* the bee, (c) *"Patti"* the Platypus, (d) *"Spinner"* or *"Web"* the Spider, (e) *"Sting"* the Ray, and (f) *"Goochie"* the Jellyfish. [NOTE: *"Hissy"* and *"Slither"* the snake are NOT clearly venomous.]

○   **In 1975, the makers of the children's toy cars called *"Hot Wheels,"* made a model named after a Ford product, called the *"Poison* [blank].*"* Fill in the [blank] with the name of the car it was named after.**

Pinto.

○   **There is a Native American dance done by members of the Arizonan *Moqui Indian* tribe, in which they danced holding what toxic critters in their mouths?**

Rattlesnakes.

○   **During the Soviet space program, they used a very dangerous rocket propellant, consisting of kerosene and liquid oxygen. It was so touchy that they gave it what diabolical toxic name?**

"Devil's Venom."

○   **In the late 1940s and early 1950s, there was a popular children's radio program called *"Straight Arrow."* The sponsor of this program produced a series of *"Straight Arrow Injun-uity Card* sets,*"* which were to be found in cereal boxes of their product. Unfortunately they had to withdraw card #19 in the series, as children were getting too close to the toxic subjects discussed to confirm their identification, and mothers thought the card was too scary and did not fit the corporate image of the company. Answer the following about this incident: (a) what was the subject of infamous, and now rare for collectors' card #19, and (b) what cereal company produced these cards?**

(a) *"Poisonous Snake Recognition,"* (b) Nabisco.

MOVIES AND TELEVISION

○ **What poison was used to murder the English professor named Dexter Cornell, played by Dennis Quaid, in the 1988 thriller movie "D.O.A."?**

Radium chloride.

○ **You have probably heard of "delta-nine THC," found in marijuana, but in what 1964 film was Ian Flemming's James Bond up against a villain that used a poisonous aerially sprayed nerve gas called "Delta-Nine"?**

"Goldfinger."

○ **In my teens I worked as a merchant seaman, where I was exposed to asbestos. I later became a Hollywood actor, well known for my action scenes on motorized vehicles. I died at the age of 50, from mesothelioma due to asbestosis. Who was I?**

Steve McQueen.

○ **What was the title of the now cult 1936 movie, which demonstrated the evils of smoking marijuana?**

"Outside in Reefer Madness."

○ **In 1926, Peggy Scott of London, England committed suicide by drinking poison. She was depressed, like many other women, over the sudden death of what widely worshiped male movie star of the silent screen?**

Rudolph Valentino.

○ **In 1990, a film was made about a deadly Venezuelan jungle spider which mates with common local Californian spiders to produce lethal offspring. What was the title of this popular movie produced by Steven Spielberg?**

"Arachnophobia."

○ **Adapted from the popular book by Michael Crichton, the 1993 movie "Jurassic Park" colorfully depicts a fictional dinosaur of toxicological significance, called the "Dilophosaur." What was its toxic nature?**

It was nicknamed *"The Spitter,"* because when it was provoked it was capable of spitting lethal venom as far as 50 feet.

❍   **What 1983 film featuring James Bond, featured a cult centered around the extremely venomous *"Blue Ringed"* Octopus?**

"Octopussy."

❍   **Television watchdog Donald Wildman, claimed that *CBS* once showed children an episode with one of their favorite cartoon heroes sniffing cocaine. What famous rodent did he finger for this apparent act of abuse?**

Mighty Mouse.

❍   **In what popular romantic 1993 movie, did the character Sam Baldwin (played by Tom Hanks), give some very good advice to the baby-sitter before leaving, by telling her where the Syrup of Ipecac was located, in case there was a poisoning emergency?**

"Sleepless in Seattle."

❍   **And now, a poisonous animal from the original Star Trek series. In the episode titled *"A Private Little War,"* Captain Kirk was bitten by a *"mugato,"* a Neuralese creature with poisonous fangs, for which there was no known antitoxin. Although Kirk was eventually successfully treated by Nona, the local *"Kahn-ut-tu"* (herbalist), who used the root of the *"mako"* plant to treat him. Describe what a *"mugato"* looked like.**

It was an apelike carnivore with white fur; red face, hands and feet; and a large horn growing out of the top of its head.

❍   **In the original series Star Trek episode *"The Man Trap,"* on planet *M113.* there is described a *"Carbon Group III vegetation, similar to the Nightshade family,"* which is mildly toxic. What was their common name of this poisonous plant?**

"Borgia plant."

❍   **In the original series Star Trek episode *"The Cloud Minders,"* a rare mineral substance was mined on the planet *"Ardana,"* which could be used to combat botanical plagues. The mineral in its raw state produced a hazardous gas which impaired mental functions, heightened emotional reactions, and stimulated violence. What was this mineral called?**

"Zenite."

❍   **In the 1992 movie *"Batman Returns,"* Batman showed his knowledge of toxic plants when he says to *Catwoman*, "[blank] *can be deadly if you eat it."* To what plant was he referring?**

Mistletoe.

❍   On April 15, 1962, the character actress Clara Blandik, age 80, died when she took an overdose of sleeping pills and put a plastic bag over her head. Her most famous movie role was as who, in what now classic 1939 film?

Auntie Em, in the *"Wizard of Oz."*

❍   On April 26, 1976, at the age of 65, the actor George Sanders, known for his roles as an urbane cad, took his own life by taking what barbiturate?

Nembutal®.

❍   On January 4, 1932, this famous American silent-screen cowboy actor, whose voice couldn't make the cut in the *"talkies,"* ended his life with cyanide in Chihuahua, Mexico. Who was he?

Art Arnold.

❍   The actor Dustin Hoffman, played a quite unique role, in a 1982 movie where his character was attempting to raise money to produce a play called *"Return to Love Canal."* What was the name of this popular movie?

"Tootsie."

❍   In 1991, a the age of 84, in a fit of depression and heavy drinking, I attempted to end my life with carbon monoxide from my automobile. In the 1950s, I was a popular father figure to millions with my series *"Father Knows Best,"* and later played the role of the ever popular Dr. Marcus Welby. What is my real name?

Robert Young.

❍   On March 5, 1982, in Los Angeles, California, what popular comedian died from an administered drug overdose when, because he was afraid of needles, a friend injected the drugs?

John Belushi.

❍   The great film director Alfred Hitchcock, once acknowledged that the infamous Crippen homicidal poisoning was his inspiration for what 1954 film starring James Stewart and Grace Kelly?

"Rear Window."

❍   Complete the following statement by filling in the blank, from the 1939 movie *"Midnight,"* when actor John Barrymore explains why a girl's parents have been worrying needlessly: *"Not measles at all. Just a simple case of* [blank] *poisoning."*

Alcohol.

❍   During the filming of the 1972 movie, *"Ciao! Manhattan,"* a medical doctor gave injections to the entire cast to maintain a high pace, and create a false sense of community. This event led to the fatal overdose of actress and model Edie Sedgwick. What drug was used?

Amphetamines.

O   What star of the 1939 movie, *"The Wizard of Oz"* began taking amphetamines to combat a weight problem, which later lead to use of barbiturates for sleep, and her eventual death from an overdose?

Judy Garland.

O   In the 1986 movie *"Little Shop of Horrors,"* Steve Martin played a sadistic dentist who meets his demise from an overdose of what substance?

Nitrous oxide, or *"Laughing gas."*

O   This movie star is famous for his battles with many exotic monsters. One such opponent was the *"Smog Monster,"* who fed from smoke stacks, and spread toxic gas over the populace of Tokyo. What is the name of the Japanese cult movie star who vanquished the toxic *"Smog Monster"*?

Godzilla.

O   In 1970, the daughter of a popular television personality, fell to her death while experiencing a severe *LSD* flashback, which resulted in her father beginning a personal crusade against drug abuse. Who was this dedicated father?

Art Linkletter.

O   *Batman* has always been known for his colorful villains. In his new cartoon show, which foe has a toxic name?

"Poison Ivy."

O   Which cult cartoon duo brought a ghost back to life by giving him a bottle of poison to drink?

Ren and Stimpy.

O   February 1991, saw some deaths on the East Coast of the United States, from heroin that had been adulterated with Methyl fentanyl, which was being sold in bags labeled with the same name as what contemporary movie title?

"Tango and Cash."

O   What famous American movie comic said he always kept some whisky handy in case he saw a snake, which he also kept handy?

W.C. Fields, *aka* Claude William Dukenfield.

❍   **What popular cartoon duo of the music world, featured episodes on toad licking and sniffing paint thinner?**

Beavis and Butthead.

❍   **In the 1956 humorous Danny Kaye movie, *"The Court Jester,"* there is a now classic scene where a *"pellet with the poison"* was placed into one of two drinking containers, and he was attempting to remember which one *NOT* to select. Was the poison in the *"vessel with the pestle,"* or the *"chalice from the palace"*?**

The vessel with the pestle.

❍   **On March 16, 1991, the actor Michael J. Fox appeared on the popular TV show *"Saturday Night Live,"* as a clown who would sting the crowd at the circus. What plant did this clown use in his act?**

The "Stinging Nettle," *Urtica dioica.*

❍   **In the television puppet show *"Rootie Kazootie,"* his arch-enemy had a rather toxic sounding name. What was it?**

"Poison Zoomack."

❍   **One has probably heard of the early, and now debunked, ptomaine theory of food poisoning. But, what 1940 Charles Chaplain movie, involved the political leaders of two countries called *"Bacteria"* and *"Tomania"*?**

"The Great Dictator."

❍   **What was the title of the 1986 movie, in which Sean Connery played the role of a monk investigating suspicious murders of fellow monks poisoned by arsenic contaminated pages of a banned book?**

"The Name of the Rose."

❍   **In the controversial 1991 movie *"My Girl,"* a young boy dies from an encounter with what toxic agent?**

Allergic reaction to bee stings.

❍   **In the popular 1989 movie *"The Bear,"* the star, a young bear cub, became intoxicated with visions after feasting on wild mushrooms. What type of mushroom was involved in the bear's meal?**

The "Fly Agaric," *Amanita muscaria muscaria.*

❍   **In the hit 1993 movie *"Sleepless in Seattle,"* a boy interrupts his father's romantic interlude by crying out that a venomous critter was in the house. Which creature did he claim to see?**

A *"Black Widow"* spider.

❍   **In one episode, the cartoon character *Homer Simpson* believed he was going to die from eating what potentially toxic dish?**

Blowfish.

❍   **What was the title of the 1986 movie which told of a nerdy janitor who fell into a barrel of toxic waste and became a hulking superhero who set out to rid the town of crime and corruption?**

"The Toxic Avenger."

❍   **What is the name of the 1963 science fiction movie, that featured plants that could walk, and kill people with their stingers?**

"Day of the Triffids."

❍   **In the 1939 movie "The Wizard of Oz," there is a reference made to poison, when the Wicked Witch of the West makes the following statement: *"And now, my beauties!...something with poison in it, I think; with poison in it, but attractive to the eye and soothing to the smell!."* Answer the following with respect to her poisonous plan to stop the travelers of the "Yellow Brick Road": (a) What was the vehicle used by the Witch to deliver her poison to the traveling foursome, (b) Who provided the antidote to save the travelers from the poison's effects? (c) What was the antidote she provided to reverse the lethargy inducing effects of the poison?**

(a) Poppies, (b) Glinda, the Good Witch of the North, (c) Falling snow.

❍   **Answer the following about a poisoning event in the 1980 comedy movie *"Airplane"*: (a) What was the contaminated food served to the passengers and crew that lead to the loss of the flying ability of *Captain Over*, the pilot, (b) What was the name of the physician on board, that tried to treat the many patients?**

(a) Fish, (b) *Dr. Rumack* (really named in honor of toxicologist Barry Rumack, by his movie producer friends).

❍   **In the 1986 movie *"Black Widow,"* starring Deborah Winger, a wife poisoned her many husbands. In what two ways was she able to administer poisons to her husbands?**

An unknown poison administered in brandy through the cork, and penicillin mixed with toothpaste to an allergic husband.

❍   **In the popular television series *"Star Trek - The Next Generation,"* the ready room of Captain Jean-Luc Picard, on the *U.S.S. Enterprise-D*, contains, a toxic decorative touch. What it is?**

An Australian *"Lionfish,"* in a saltwater wall-aquarium.

❍   **What was the name of the 1973 horror movie, in which Strother Martin plays a doctor who finds a way of transforming man into a deadly** *"King Cobra"*?

"Sssssss."

❍   **He was a superhero with the colorful name of a toxic critter. His real identity was Britt Reid (the great grand-nephew of** *"The Lone Ranger"*). **Who was his superhero persona?**

"The Green Hornet."

❍   **This 1945 movie which won the** *Academy Award* **for best picture and best actor saw Ray Milland realistically portraying the chronic toxic effects of alcohol on the human system. What was the title of this classic film?**

"The Lost Weekend."

❍   **In a 1971 movie, the destitute playboy Henry Graham (played by Walter Matthau), plans to marry and kill a wealthy but clumsy botanist, and in the film he is seen studying a book titled** *Beginner's Guide to Toxicology*. **What is the name of this film?**

"A New Leaf."

❍   **The 1979 film** *"Prophecy,"* **directed by John Frankenheimer, tells of bears in a national park, which due to environmental contamination turn into hideous monsters that prey on unsuspecting campers. What toxic substance in their environment caused this terrible change?**

Mercury.

❍   **In this 1967 movie, James Bond, as a cover is married to a Japanese girl diver who is tragically poisoned while sleeping by a Ninja assassin working for** *SPECTRE*. **What is the title of this film?**

"You Only Live Twice."

❍   **In February 1995, a popular television soap opera showed a wife, Gloria Chandler, poisoning her husband Adam by placing arsenic in his food. What is the name of this popular soap opera?**

"All My Children."

❍   **In the movies** *"Raiders of the Lost Ark,"* **Indiana Jones has to enter a chamber filled with snakes. What type of snakes does his friend say they are?**

Asps.

❍   **What popular 1980 movie saw inhabitants of a tropical island, dealing with such toxic agents as a** *"Stone Fish"* **and the seeds of** *Abrus precatorius*?

"The Blue Lagoon."

❍   **In 1995, a movie staring Hugh O'Connor was released titled *"The Young Poisoner's Handbook,"* which was based on the life of what notorious British homicidal poisoner?**

Graham Frederick Young.

❍   **In what hit movie do Jim Carrey and Cameron Diaz admire how methane sets off the color of a sunset?**

"The Mask."

❍   **In the movie *"Jurassic Park,"* scientists investigate the poisoning of a dinosaur by the *"West Indian Lilac"* plant. What type of dinosaur was the suspected victim?**

A Triceratops.

❍   **In the made for television movie *"The Black Widow Murders: The Blanche Taylor Moore Story,"* what actress played the role of the title character?**

Elizabeth Montgomery.

❍   **The actor Joe Pesci starred *"With Honors,"* a 1994 movie about a bum who went to Harvard. His character dies at the end due to the effects of being exposed years before to what toxic substance?**

Asbestos.

❍   **In an episode of the popular cartoon show *"The Simpsons,"* Bart takes a trip to France on an exchange program, where he is enslaved by a couple of nasty vintners, and is forced to drink some adulterated wine. What was the adulterant in the wine?**

Antifreeze.

❍   **A 1994 comedy movie begins when a musician dies from arsenic laced booze. Later another murder occurs by the use of Nitrous oxide. The film involves employees at station *WBN*, surrounded by murders as they prepare for their first national radio broadcast. What was the name of this popular film?**

"Radioland Murders."

❍   **In the 1976 movie *"Robin and Marion,"* with Sean Connery and Audrey Hepburn, Robin and Marion both die at the end from drinking from a poisoned cup. Who was the poisoner?**

Maid Marion herself. It was a homicide/suicide act.

❍   **What popular 1940 Disney film had mushrooms dancing to Tchaikovsky's *"Nutcracker Suite"*?**

"Fantasia."

❍   The title of what Oscar winning 1973 film, about a well executed con game, sounds very much like what might happen if you had caught a member of genus *Bombus* in your hand?

"The Sting."

❍   In the early days of movie special effects, what toxic substance was used on the set to create artificial clouds and fog, before its use was banned?

Carbon tetrachloride.

❍   In the popular 1981, film *"Clash of the Titans,"* Perseus battles giant venomous creatures that spring from the blood of Medusa. What type of creatures did he battle?

Scorpions.

❍   In the popular 1995 movie *"Waterworld,"* a scene shows the leading character played by Kevin Costner, eating what plant's leaves considered toxic by those in the know?

Tomato, *Lycopersicum esculentum.*

❍   What is the title of the 1996 thriller film, which tells the story of a former prison inmate (Sean Connery) and an *FBI* agent (Nicholas Cage), who team up to save San Francisco from a terrorist planned poison gas attack, launched from Alcatraz?

"The Rock."

❍   What was the title of the 1993 movie about mosquitos that have been contaminated with toxic waste, turning them into huge, winged blood suckers, that attack a town?

"Skeeter."

❍   What was the title of the 1970 film, that depicted young people inheriting the earth after a chemical is released that kills everyone over 30 years of age?

"Gas-s-s-s."

❍   In 1991, the television movie *"Wife, Mother, Murderer,"* staring Judith Light, told the story of an infamous Alabama poisoner? Who's events were chronicled in this drama?

Audrey Marie Hilley.

❍   **The Victorian story of a dysfunctional family turning to murder was told in a *"Masterpiece Theater"* adaptation of a 1978 novel by Julian Symons. What was the name of this dark presentation?**

"The Blackheath Poisonings."

❍   **Which popular cast member of the TV show *"Frasier"* nearly died on the set from an overdose of rat poison?**

"Moose," the Jack Russell terrier who plays *"Eddie."*

❍   **In an easily forgettable film, Suzanne Somers plays a vacationer overwhelmed by an unstoppable army of very toxic ants. What was the name of this movie?**

"Ants."

❍   **On the popular TV show *"Seinfeld,"* George's fiancee is poisoned and dies. How did this tragedy happen?**

From licking engagement envelopes having a toxic glue.

❍   **The plot of an episode of this popular television space adventure involved the conflict of two member of the *"Q" continuum*, one of which wanted to commit suicide. He eventually died after ingesting a *"Nogatch Hemlock"* plant. On what series did this toxicological episode occur?**

"Star Trek Voyager."

❍   **What actor plays Stanley Goodspeed, a toxic chemicals specialist for the *FBI*, in the 1996, thriller *"The Rock"*?**

Nicholas Cage.

❍   **In what 1991 movie did Dustin Hoffman play a pirate who punished one of his crewman by locking him in a chest, then dropping black scorpions in with him?**

"Hook."

❍   **What Broadway hit deals with a convent whose numbers were depleted after being served Botulism tainted Vichyssoise soup?**

"Nunsense."

❍   **What 1996 action thriller film, starring actor Kurt Russell, involved a group of terrorists who take over a *747* airliner, with a toxic plan to bomb the United States, with stolen Soviet *"DZ-5"* nerve gas?**

"Executive Decision."

○   **Alcoholics are known to often turn to other alcohols for relief, and in what 1966 film featuring Richard Burton and Elizabeth Taylor, as a couple of battling alcoholics, does one hear the line *"Martha? Rubbing alcohol for you?"***

"Who's Afraid of Virginia Woolf?"

○   **In what 1987, film did the character Owen Lifts (played by Danny DeVito), try to kill his overbearing mother by adding lye to her soft drink?**

"Throw Mama from the Train ."

○   **The 1973 film *"And Millions Will Die,"* centers around a madman who has buried a time bomb filled with toxic nerve gas beneath the streets of what populated Asian city?**

Hong Kong.

○   **What was the title of the 1996 film, with Dan Akroyd and Jack Lemon, which involved an ethics professor who poisons the apples on the tree of a neighbor everyone believes is a fugitive Nazi war criminal, only to find he has made a tragic error?**

"Getting Away With Murder."

○   **What 1994 film, involved the murder of a private detective with strychnine, and a widow and a cop investigating the murder of a Beverly Hills couple?**

"Perfect Alibi."

○   **What 1997 film, involved a policeman trying to stop a psychopath from poisoning Chicago's water supply?**

"Lethal Tender."

○   **In the 1949 film *"Prince of Foxes,"* Orson Wells portrayed what infamous Renaissance poisoner?**

Cesare Borgia.

○   **What was the title of the 1934 suspense film, staring Charles Starrett, Edward Van Sloan, and Shirley Grey, which told of a madman killing students with poison gas?**

"Murder on the Campus."

○   **What is the title of the 1996 film, which centers around a pharmaceutical company's attempt to develop an antidote to counteract the nationwide blissful catatonia resulting from the premature release of an untested antidepressant to the public?**

"Kids in the Hall Brain Candy."

❍   **A 1997 episode of this popular television series involved an inventive poisoner who used toxic creatures to murder rich people, then taunted the *VCTF* with clues. What is the name of the series?**

"Profiler."

❍   **In the 1995 film *"The Net,"* Sandra Bullock's boyfriend was murdered by what method, in an attempt to cover up the computer plot she was caught up in?**

His medications were switched resulting in an allergic response to penicillin.

❍   **In the movie *"Matilda,"* starring Danny DeVito and Rhea Perlman, they played parents with the same toxic name as the plant that is used to produce *"Absinthe."* What was their family name?**

The *Wormwoods*.

❍   **What actress on the sitcom *"Wings"* had to be treated with hyperbaric Oxygen (*HBO*), after being poisoned by Carbon monoxide, while she was in her trailer on the set?**

Crystal Bernard.

❍   **What little blue cartoon characters live inside a *"Fly Agaric"* mushroom?**

Smurfs.

❍   **Finnish film maker Aki Kaurismaki, in his 1993 film, tells the story of Iris, who turns from being a worn-out drudge into a serial poisoner, who gets back at everyone who had ever abused her. What is the title of this camp humor film?**

"The Match Factory Girl."

❍   **In this 1996, comedy film, five graduate students begin to eliminate right winged dinner guests weekly, by serving them Arsenic laced wine. What was the title of this film?**

"The Last Supper."

❍   **In the 1939 film the *"Wizard of Oz,"* the role of the Tin Man was originally to be played by Buddy Ebsen, but he was eventually replaced by actor Jack Haley, because Buddy suffered what toxic reaction?**

He had a severe respiratory reaction to the powdered Aluminum dust used in the Tinman makeup.

❍   **In the *1954 classic, "Creature from the Black Lagoon,"* what toxic substance was placed in the water to capture the "gill-man" creature?**

Rotenone.

○ **A 1994 British television program titled *"Dandelion Dead,"* told the true story of a henpecked wife-poisoner, From Hay-on-Wye, Wales, who in 1921, became the first solicitor hanged in Britain. Who was he?**

Herbert Rowse Armstrong.

○ **In 1944, Charles Laughten starred in a film titled *"The Suspect,"* which was based on what famous British poisoner?**

Dr. Harley Harvey Crippen.

○ **Because the general public is both fascinated and fearful of poisonous things, movie creators have often use larger than life themes in creating horror and science fiction movies. Given a very short description, give the exact title of the following films: (a) The 1954 film which featured radiation generated giant ants, (b) The 1955 film which featured a biologically generated giant spider, (c) The 1957 film which featured a giant arachnid which came from a Mexican volcano, (d) The 1958 film which featured, mutated wasps from a mission in space?**

(a) *"Them!,"* (b) *"Tarantula,"* (c) *"The Black Scorpion,"* (d) *"The Monster From the Green Hell."*

○ **Because the general public is both fascinated and fearful of poisonous things, movie creators have often used larger than life themes in creating horror and science fiction movies. Given a very short description, give the exact title of the following films: (a) The 1959 film which featured a large *Heloderma*, terrorizing the Southwest, (b) The 1959 film which featured an island populated by large venomous shrews, (c) The 1963 film which featured a group of people shipwrecked on an island, who eat a fungus and are transformed into fungal creatures, (d) The 1954 film which featured a Brazilian plantation owner fighting an army of venomous red ants, called *"Marabunta."***

(a) *"The Giant Gila Monster,"* (b) *"The Killer Shrews,"* (c) *"Attack of the Mushroom People,"* (d) *"The Naked Jungle."*

○ **Many of the Spielberg movies about the adventures of Indiana Jones, have featured poisons in the plots. Give the complete title of the film which depicted the following: (a) Indiana attempts to chase a bottle of antidote for the poison he has been given, across a nightclub's crowded dance floor, (b) An attempt is made to get the hero, by using poisoned dates, but the attempt was thwarted by a monkey's intervention.**

(a) *"Indiana Jones and the Temple of Doom"* (1984), *(b) "Raiders of the Lost Ark"* (1981).

○ **Give the title of each of following movies in which the actor's dialogue involved the theme of poisons: (a) *"For a gallon of elderberry wine, I take one teaspoonful of*** *arsenic, then add a half teaspoon of strychnine and then just a pinch of cyanide.", (b) "Oh, I see...the pellet with the poison's in the flagon with the dragon; the vessel with the pestle has the brew that is true.", (c) "Back where I come from, folks call that love stuff a quick poison, it hurts you all over real bad, like a shot of electricity. But if it's slow poison, well it's like a fever that aches in your bones for a thousand years.", (d) "The one without the parsley is the one without the poison.", (e) "I'd hate to take a bite out of you. You're a cookie full of arsenic."?*

(a) *"Arsenic and Old Lace"* (1944), (b) *"The Court Jester"* (1956), (c) *"A Guy Named Joe"* (1943), (d) *"Roman Scandals"* (1933), (e) *"Sweet Smell of Success"* (1957).

○   **This 1980 film told the story of three lady office workers who think they accidentally gave their nasty boss rat poison instead of the sweetener *"Skinny and Sweet."* What was the name of the popular film?**

"Nine to Five."

○   **In this popular 1980 film, Lloyd Bridges, as a harried air controller says, *"Looks like I picked the wrong week to quit amphetamines...Looks like I picked the wrong week to quit sniffing glue."* What was the name of this hilarious film?**

"Airplane."

○   **In the Three Stooges classic film *"Disorder in the Court,"* Larry mistakes a man's toupee for what venomous creature?**

A tarantula.

○   **The actor Tom Cruise is often cast in the role of an attorney. In a 1992 film, he is asked to defend two marines accused of poisoning one of their comrades. Answer the following about this film: (a) What was the name of this film, (b) How was the poison administered, and (c) What was the poison?**

(a) *"A Few Good Men,"* (b) A soaked rag placed in the victim's mouth, (c) The poison was never identified.

○   **David Bowie, Dennis Hopper, and Gary Oldman, all made cameo roles in the film about this graffiti artist who died in 1988 of a cocaine and heroin overdose. Who was this famous artist?**

Jean M. Basquiat.

○   **In the TV sitcom series *"Friends,"* Monica is stung by a jellyfish. How did Chandler treat her sting?**

By urinating upon it.

○   **In what 1987 popular film, was there a duel of wits between the Dread Pirate Roberts and the kidnapper Vizzini using *"Iocane"* powder placed in a wine goblet?**

"The Princess Bride."

○   In this *"I Love Lucy"* classic episode, Lucy suffers the toxic effects of taking too many doses of an elixir while making a commercial. What was the name of this product which contained 28% ethanol?

"Vita-meata-vegamin."

○   In the 1976 Alfred Hitchcock film *Family Plot*, what sedative drug was used to subdue the kidnap victim?

Ketamine.

○   What action film of 1997, involved a computer engineer suffering from copper poisoning, who takes over and tries to destroy, a cruise ship in order to steal diamonds, and get back for being discharged by his employers?

"Speed 2 – Cruise Control."

○   What was the title of the popular crime spoof movie containing the line: *"Cops and women don't mix. It's like swallowing a spoonful of Drano^R. Sure, it'll clean you out, but it leaves you feeling hollow inside."*?

"Naked Gun."

○   In Keenan and Kel's movie *"Good Burger,"* a poison for killing what creatures was placed in the secret sauce?

Sharks.

○   In what Disney movie can you hear the line *"Drown them, poison them, bash them on the head. Got any chloroform? I don't care how you kill the little beasts, just do it!,"* being delivered by actress Glen Close?

"101 Dalmatians."

○   In what Disney film, does actor Chris O'Donnel say *"As morning hues of sunswept fire caress your poisoned face..."*?

"The 3 Musketeers."

○   A popular sitcom which aired on November 5, 1951, depicted a harrowed housewife who had been reading too many *Mockingbird Murder Mysteries*, and thought her husband would try to kill her by methods including poisoning. What was the name of this show in which the lady said *"I got a Micky from Ricky"*?

"I Love Lucy."

❍   In the 1966, Hitchcock Cold War thriller, *Torn Curtain*, with Paul Newman by what improbable toxic means does he kill his attacker, during the fight in the kitchen?

By putting his head in a gas oven.

❍   What famous comedic actor said the following to Carlotta Monti: *"Never cry over spilt milk, because it may have been poisoned."*?

W. C. Fields.

❍   What is the name of the 1957 movie that tells the story of a man who was accidentally sprayed with a toxic pesticide which caused him to slowly decrease in size to almost nothing?

"The Incredible Shrinking Man."

❍   In 1998 there was a film, which involved a gene spliced combination of a Cobra and an Eastern Diamondback, which was over 30 feet long? In this film actor Pat Morita played the knowledgeable herpetologist. What was the name of this thriller film?

"King Cobra."

❍   This very popular 1983 television science-fiction series tells of the fight between earthlings and alien visitors who threaten to establish a Fascist dictatorship. The aliens are eventually defeated by the defender's use of a poisonous *"red dust."* What was the name of this intriguing series?

"V."

❍   In a episode of *"All in the Family,"* Archie Bunker received what antidote when he believed he had eaten a can of *"persined" Bronco Brand* mushrooms?

Botulinus Antitoxin.

❍   In a classic *Bugs Bunny* episode, *Bugs* was captured by *Witch Hazel*, but not chopped up because he reminded her of her toxic pet *"Paul."* What kind of pet was *"Paul"*?

Tarantula.

❍   On January 19, 1996, the producer of the popular movies *"Top Gun,"* and *"Flash Dance,"* died from an overdose of a mixture of *"Speed"* and wine. Who was he?

Don Simpson.

◯　**On January 29, 1964, this popular male actor of the 1940s and 1950s, who starred in the 1953 movie *"Shane,"* committed suicide with sedatives and alcohol. Who was he?**

Alan Ladd.

MUSIC

○ **In the Rodgers and Hammerstein popular musical *"The Sound of Music,"* Maria sings a song titled *"My Favorite Things."* In this song is a reference to a venomous animal. What animal is it?**

The bee. *"When the dog bites, when the bee stings..."*

○ **The untimely death of what famous singer, from bulemia, jeopardized the *OTC* sale of Syrup of Ipecac?**

Karen Carpenter.

○ **During the 1960s, the *Jefferson Airplane* sang a popular song dealing with hallucinogenic drugs. Can you name this song which began with the following lyrics: *"One pill makes you larger, and one pill makes you small. And the ones that mother gives you don't do anything at all. Go ask Alice, when she's ten feet tall..."*?**

"White Rabbit."

○ **In 1791, a famous musician died and poisoning was suspected. Later, one of his chief musical rivals, Antonio Salieri, is reported to have confessed to poisoning him. Who was this famous composer?**

Wolfgang Amadeus Mozart.

○ **This 1968 rock musical had references in it to the hallucinogen *"STP."* What was the name of this musical?**

"Hair."

○ **We all know it can be dangerous to mix alcohol with sedatives. In June 1953, a famous Country singer mixed booze with chloral hydrate and was found dead in the back of his limousine, in Oak Ridge, West Virginia. His last song was *"I'll Never Get Out of this World Alive."* Who was he?**

Hank Williams.

○ **It has almost been proven that a great Italian violinist, unrivaled in virtuosity, who lived from 1782-1840, succumbed from medical treatments he had received with mercury. Who was this great musician?**

Nicolo Paganini.

O   **Heavy use of cocaine can cause perforation of the nasal septum. What member of the 1960s popular band *"Crosby, Stills, Nash, and Young,"* admitted to suffering from this condition?**

David Crosby.

O   **Poisons have figured in many an opera plot. But in which of the following operas was the poisoning feigned and NOT actually taken: Puccini's *"Tosca,"* Puccini's *"Sugor Angelica,"* "Mozart's *"Cosi Fan Tutti,"* Verdi's *"Il Trovatore,"* or Wagner's *"Tristan and Isolde"*?**

Mozart's *"Cosi Fan Tutti."*

O   **The death of what famous rock music entertainer, in 1977, was hastened by use of opiates and tranquilizers?**

Elvis Presley.

O   **In 1988, a famous musician was arrested and charged with driving under the influence of *PCP*. He is often called the *"Godfather of Soul,"* but what's the real name of this personage?**

James Joe Brown Jr.

O   **In the 1930s, a famous Blues singer named Robert Johnson was murdered. What plant was implicated in the cause of death?**

"Jimson Weed," *Datura stramonium.*

O   **A famous western song featured the lyrics *"the longhorn cattle feed on the lowly Jimson Weed...."* Answer the following about this song: (a) What western singer made this song famous? (b) What was the title of this song?**

(a) Gene Autry, (b) *"Back in the Saddle Again."*

O   **In an 1865 opera by Jacob Mayerbeer dealing with the adventures of the Portuguese explorer Vasco da Gama, a young lover commits suicide by eating the poisonous flowers of a tree. Answer the following about his opera: (a) What is identity of the mythical tree? (b) What is the name of the opera?**

(a) Manzanillo, (b) *"L'Africaine."*

O   **In the early part of the 20th century, a popular song contained the lyrics *"I get no kick from cocaine — I'm sure that if I took even one sniff, It would bore me terrifically, too...."* Answer the following about this song: (a) Name the composer. (b) What is the title of this piece?**

(a) Cole Porter, (b) *"I Get a Kick Out of You."*

⃝   I am a famous singer of children's songs and one of my more popular tunes was about a little whale. I gave up children's songs in recent years and became an environmental singer when I learned that the whales I sang about swim in a river so polluted that when they are beached, their whale carcasses are treated as toxic waste. Answer the following about me: (a) What is my name? (b) What is the common name of these whales? (c) What is the name of the polluted river?

(a) Raffi, (b) Beluga, (c) St. Lawrence River.

⃝   Name the artist or artists who performed each of the following songs that have a toxic reference in the song title: (a) *"Poison Ivy,"* (b) *"Poison,"* (c) *"Shot of Poison,"* (d) *"Lithium."*

(a) The Coasters, (b) Bel Biv Devoe, (c) Lita Ford, (d) Nirvana.

⃝   Name the artist or artists who performed each of the following songs that have a toxic reference in the song title: (a) *"Cocaine,"* (b) *"The Acid Queen,"* (c) *"Sister Morphine,"* (d) *"The Sidewinder Sleeps."*

(a) Eric Clapton, (b) *"The Who,"* (c) *"The Rolling Stones,"* (d) *"REM."*

⃝   In this opera by Ralph Vaughan Williams, the character *Tormentilla* eventually marries a shepherd boy, who is actually a Prince in disguise. Because *Tormentilla* is immune to all poisons, the attempts of the Empress to stop the relationship are thwarted. What is the name the opera which tells this fantastic toxicologic story?

"The Poisoned Kiss."

⃝   Donizetti wrote an opera which tells the story of a supposed real poisoner, who in actuality probably never poisoned anyone. What was the name of this opera?

"Lucrezia Borgia."

⃝   The Russian composer Nikolai Andreevich Rimsky-Korsakov (1844-1908), composed a classic piece of music about a venomous creature. What is the name of his popular composition?

"Flight of the Bumblebee."

⃝   *"The Banana Boat Song"* made popular in the 1960s by the singer Harry Belafonte, mentions in the lyrics, a secretive toxic critter. What is this animal?

A Tarantula. *"...hides the deadly Black Tarantula..."*

⃝   In the 1960s, with lyrics like *"when they see us coming...all try an' hide, but they still go for peanuts when coated with cyanide"* and *"my pulse will be quickenin' with each drop of strychnine,"* satirical lyricist Tom Leher, wrote a song about poisoning what kind of animal in what location?

"Poisoning Pigeons In The Park."

◯   **Name the artist who in his 1978 album *"Squeezing Out Sparks,"* had a hit single titled *"Mercury Poisoning"*?**

Graham Parker and the Rumour.

◯   **The strains of a dance featuring quick hops and foot-tapping music can be heard in the creations of such composers as Chopin, Liszt, and Tchaikovsky. This music style descended directly from what Italian folk-dance associated with a toxic entity?**

The *"Tarantella,"* associated with spider bites.

◯   **On July 2, 1971, what famous rock star supposedly died in a Paris apartment, from an overdose of heroin?**

Jim Morrison (1943-1971).

◯   **In 1961, a musical was produced, written by Wolf Mankowitz, which starred George Benson as an infamous British poisoner. It was titled *"Belle, or the Ballad of* [blank]." What poisoner's activities were set to music?**

Dr. Crippen (Hawley Harvey Crippen).

◯   **The best selling music album of 1995, was made by a band with the name which sounds like a toxic animal. What is the name of the popular band?**

"Hootie and the Blowfish."

◯   **In which rock opera, does the title character sing, *"I just want to say...if there is a way...take this cup away from me...I don't want to taste it's poison..."*?**

"Jesus Christ Superstar."

◯   **In Francesco Cilea's opera, *"Adriana Lecouvreur,"* the heroine smells a bunch of poisoned flowers and dies after suffering spasms and delirium. What type of flowers had been poisoned?**

Violets.

◯   **In the Rodgers and Hammerstein musical *"South Pacific,"* one can hear the sailors singing about a character named *"Bloody Mary,"* who practices the art of abusing what plant substance?**

"Betel Nut," *Areca catechu.*

◯   **This 1997 pop music combo from San Francisco, California, with songs such as *"Sail the Black Seas," "Kiss Me, You Fool!,"* and *"The Artful Ventriloquist,"* goes by a toxic name related to the historical use of arsenic in chronic doses to carry out homicides. What is the name of this musical group?**

"The Slow Poisoners."

○   **What famous Italian singer spent years paying extortion to the *"Black Hand"* criminal organization, who threatened to harm him by putting Lye into his drink to ruin his voice, should payments of 10% of his performance fees be stopped?**

Enrico Caruso (1873-1921).

○   **Some people enjoy "heavy metal" music. Complete the name of each of the following musical groups or personalities, with the appropriate toxic metallic substance: (a) _____ *Zeplin*, (b) _____ *Maiden*, (c) *Freddy* _____, (d) _____ *Butterfly*.**

(a) Lead, *sic Led*, (b) *Iron*, (c) Mercury, (d) *Iron*.

○   **Alan Jackson must come from the toxicological school of romance. In his hit song *"There Goes...,"* he describes the woman he loves as what venomous creature?**

A Black Widow spider.

○   **What music group with the name of a *Hymenoptera*, was nominated in 1999, for a *Grammy Award* for jazz?**

Yellowjackets.

○   **Barely four feet tall, Thomas Quasthoff is one of Germany's most acclaimed bass-baritones. What toxic event caused the condition that inspired one spiteful critic to label him a *"gnome"*?**

Born in 1960, Quasthoff was a Thalidomide baby.

○   **In the Jimmy Buffet sone *"Volcano,"* he sings he doesn't want to land in what toxic place because he doesn't want *"to see my skin a'glow"*?**

Three Mile Island.

○   **In 1999, many people protested a song released by a singing group, that told of the poisoning murder by a girl named Wanda, of her physically abusive husband. (a) What was the name of the singing group?, (b) What was the title of the song?, and (c) What was the title of their CD which contained the song?**

(a) *Dixie Chicks*, (b) *"Goodbye Earl,"* (c) *"FLY."*

○   **Who was the Tennessee reared Queen of Country Music who, when a child, her father pulled her from a church where she was singing when the preacher behind her started to handle a poisonous snake?**

Dolly Parton.

PERSONAGES

❍   In April, 1989, 1960s activist and founder of the *"Yippie"* movement, Abbie Hoffman, was found dead in his home in New Hope, Pennsylvania. His death was ruled a suicide by an overdose of what drug along with alcohol?

Phenobarbital.

❍   Lady Astor, who was known for her quick wit and sharp tongue, is supposed to have said to a gentleman seated next to her at dinner: *"If you were my husband...I'd put poison in your tea,"* to which the gentleman quickly replied: *"and if I were your husband, I'd drink it."* Who was the famous and equally quick witted gentleman?

Sir Winston Churchill.

❍   In January 1975, Mitsugoro Bando *VIII*, one of Japan's most gifted Kabuki actors, and a living *"national treasure,"* died from poisoning after eating in a Kyoto restaurant. What did he consume that poisoned him?

Fugu (puffer fish) liver, containing tetrodotoxin.

❍   In the 1960s, the *CIA* concocted a plan to poison Fidel Castro of Cuba. By what means did they plan to deliver the poison?

By poisoning his cigars.

❍   We know that exposure to excessive amounts of radiation can have toxic consequences, but who was the first person known to have died of radiation exposure?

Madame Marie Curie.

❍   What famous physician was so enthralled by the effects of cocaine that he published a work titled *Uber Coca*?

Sigmund Freud.

❍   Upon the death of this United States President in August 1923, rumors abounded that he had been poisoned by his wife, Florence Kling DeWolfe, because of his marital infidelities. Who was he?

Warren G. Harding.

O   She was called the *"World's Most Pulchritudinous Evangelist,"* and was the founder in 1926 of the *International Institute of Four-Square Evangelism.* She died in 1944, from an overdose of sleeping pills. Who was this once famous woman?

Sister Aimee Semple McPhearson.

O   In 1915, the German chemist Fritz Haber, developed what was known as the *"ct product."* His formula was *c x t = a constant.* Toxicologically what did all this mean?

The product of the concentration of the poison and the survival time is a constant.

O   Her name was Isabel Rosario Cooper (also known as *"Dimples"*), and she committed suicide in 1960, by taking an overdose of barbiturates. Before their romance ended, she had been the long time mistress of what famous American military figure of World Wars I, II, and Korea?

General Douglas McArthur.

O   If one were to review the medical history of President George Bush, one would find he has an allergy to what toxic agent?

Bee venom.

O   What military personage after serving as President of the United States, wrote his memoirs while taking large amounts of cocaine, for the treatment of his terminal illness?

Ulysses S. Grant.

O   On October 31, 1993, outside a music club called the *"Viper Room"* in West Hollywood, California, a toxic combination of cocaine and opiates, caused the death of what popular, drug abusing, 23-year-old actor?

River Phoenix.

O   Such notables of the day as: Sir Humphrey Davy, Samuel Taylor Coleridge, Robert Southey, and Peter Roget, gathered at parties to abuse by inhalation, what newly discovered anesthetic substance?

Nitrous oxide.

O   In London, England, on September 23, 1939, this famous psychologist who was plagued by oral cancer from smoking 20 cigars a day was administered a fatal dose of morphine by his physician for euthanasia. Who was this famous patient?

Dr. Sigmund Freud.

○   **Intoxication by lead in the production of his white pigments, has been attributed to have caused symptoms of lead encephalopathy in what famous Spanish painter, who lived from 1746-1828?**

"Goya," or Francisco Jose de Goya y Lucientes.

○   **On September 12, 1991, 65 year old Adan Garza of McAllen, Texas, became a toxicological first in the United States, when he came in contact with what toxicological entities?**

"Africanized Killer Bees," when he suffered over 300 stings, in the first major documented attack in the United States.

○   **On June 6, 1799, in the State of Virginia, a great American patriot died when in an attempt to cure his illness, he was given a dose of poisonous mercury. This remedy denied him of his liberty and gave him death. Who was he?**

Patrick Henry.

○   **While exploring New Caledonia in 1774, the Captain of the *HMS Resolution*, nearly died from tetrodotoxin poisoning. What was the name of this illustrious nautical explorer?**

Capt. James Cook.

○   **In the 1970s a case was made that Napoleon had been poisoned during his internment on the island of St. Helena. What poison was implicated in his death?**

Arsenic.

○   **If the *"Rugely Poisoner"* were to meet the French *"Black Widow,"* who would be meeting whom, of homicidal poisoners?**

William Palmer, M.D. (1855) would meet Marie Besnard (1949).

○   **We know that petroleum hydrocarbons are pervasive throughout society and can be toxic, but what popular humorist said *"We are the first nation in the history of the world to go to the Poorhouse in an automobile."***

Will Rogers.

○   **In 1980, after Los Angeles attorney Paul Morantz won a $300,000 settlement against the drug rehabilitation center *Synanon* for holding a woman captive in the 1970s, *Synanon* leader Charles Dederich attempted to murder the lawyer by putting what toxic agent in his mailbox?**

A 54 inch diamond back rattlesnake, which bit the victim's thumb.

❍   In 1973, Karen Silkwood died in a mysterious car accident at the same time she was trying to expose the *Kerr-McGee Corporation* of contaminating their work environment with what toxic material?

Plutonium.

❍   In 1888 a pharmacist by the name of John S. Pemberton developed something he called *"Esteemed Brain Tonic and Intellectual Beverage"* which contained: caffeine, secret ingredients, and cocaine. Modified for use today, by what better name do we know this product?

Coca Cola® .

❍   In the 1980s, what veteran evangelist was hospitalized from the bite of a *"Brown Recluse"* spider?

Rev. Billy Graham.

❍   King Charlemagne of France used to dazzle his dinner guests by throwing his napkin into the fire and retrieving it cleaned and intact. Out of what material, now considered hazardous, was his napkin made?

Asbestos.

❍   In England, around 1531, Richard Roose, the chef of the Bishop of Rochester, was convicted of poisoning the household with a meat sauce seasoned with hemlock and deadly nightshade. He was given a place in history by being the first criminal executed in England by what newly made legal method?

Being boiled alive.

❍   On what important type of antidotes used in toxicology did the following men do early research: Henry Sewell (1887) of Michigan, and Albert Calmette (1895) of Paris, France?

Antivenins.

❍   In 1898, this famous French post-impressionist painter attempted suicide, unsuccessfully, by taking arsenic. Known for his paintings of South Pacific native scenes, he is buried in the Marquesses islands. Who was he?

Paul Gauguin (1848-1903).

❍   What former U.S. First Lady with a long-running addiction to alcohol and drugs, later underwent successful rehabilitation?

Betty Ford.

❍   Name the mayor of Washington, D.C., who was arrested in 1989, for use of crack cocaine, and was later convicted only for cocaine possession?

Mayor Marion Barry.

❍   **In 1912, pharmacologist Wilbur Scoville devised the *"Scoville Organoleptic Test"* for measuring the relative power of what irritating principle, that is also a component of ethnic recipes world wide?**

Capsaicin, the irritant principle of the chile pepper.

❍   **In 1829, what contribution to toxicology was made by Drs. Thomas Addison and John Morgan?**

They wrote the first book in English on the action of poisons on the living body.

❍   **Charles John Samuel (C.J.S.) Thompson (1863-1943), was one of the honorary curators at the *Museum of the Royal College of Surgeons* in England. What was his contribution to the study of poisons?**

He authored some of the first books discussing the romance and history of poisons and poisonings.

❍   **In 1991, John Linner, a Houston scientist was accused of attempting to poison a co-worker by administering the carcinogenic compound *beta-propiolactone*. What was the chosen method of administration?**

The chemical was placed in the victim's nasal spray.

❍   **In 1991, a famous American military and political personage was exhumed, to check for the possibility of death due to arsenic poisoning. Having died in 1850, shortly after espousing anti-slavery views, this person is buried in Louisville, Kentucky. No arsenic was found, but who was this famous individual?**

Zachary Taylor, 12th American President.

❍   **Sir Max Beerbohm was referring to whom when he wrote: *"I maintain that though you would often in the fifteenth century have heard the snobbish Roman say, in a would-be off-hand tone, 'I am dining with the* [blank] *tonight,' no Roman was able to say, 'I dined last night with the* [blank]'."?**

Borgias.

❍   **Who was the social satirist and foulmouthed humorist of the 1950s and 1960s, who died from a self-administered overdose of morphine?**

Lenny Bruce (1925-1966).

❍   **The Italian, Bernardino Ramazzini (1633-1714), published a treatise titled *De Morbisi Artificium Diatriba*. What was the significance of his contributions to toxicology?**

He was probably the first to undertake the careful study of the disease of workers, based on direct observations of the workers and the workplaces.

○   **Finally discovered in Tulsa, Oklahoma, in 1954, Nannie Doss had poisoned eleven family members over a period of 30 years. By what popular name was she known in the press of the time?**

"Arsenic Annie."

○   **Socialite Claus von Bulow was accused of trying to kill his wife *"Sunny"* in 1980 by what means?**

Insulin injection.

○   **It has been speculated that the artist Vincent VanGogh's symptoms of anorexia, nausea, yellow-green vision, and hallucinations, were due to intoxication by what drug he may have received while institutionalized at the *Asylum of St. Paul*, at St. Remey, France, around 1888?**

Digitalis lanata.

○   **American dentist, Horace Wells, was the first person in the United States to use nitrous oxide in surgery. He died from complications resulting from his own chronic abuse of what substance?**

Chloroform.

○   **George Qythe, an original signer of the *Declaration of Independence,* was murdered by his nephew. What toxic substance was placed in his coffee and on strawberries eaten by Mr. Wythe and his family?**

Arsenic.

○   **Which of the twelve apostles is also the patron saint against poisons?**

St. John the Evangelist (or the *Apostle,* or the *Beloved*).

○   **This English king was rumored to have died, when a monk squeezed toad toxins into his wine. Being Richard the *"Lion-Hearted's"* villainous brother in the tales of Robin Hood, he is mostly associated with the *Magna Carta*. Who was he?**

King John I (John "Lackland" Plantagenet).

○   **The 17th century physician Eberhard Gockel, wrote treatises on how to cure the medical consequences of encounters with witches and werewolves. But, his toxicological claim to fame was the discovery of an assay to detect an adulterant placed in wine, and that this adulterant caused illness. What was the toxic adulterant?**

Lead.

❍   The following personages all are said to have died from the ingestion of what poisonous source: Pope Clement *VII*, the Emperor Jovian, the Emperor Charles *VI*, Berronill of Naples, and the widow of Tsar Alexis?

Mushrooms.

❍   In 1840, the French woman Marie Lafarge was convicted of murdering her husband through the use of what new analytical test?

"Marsh Test."

❍   In 1990, a pathologist named Jack Kervorkian, M.D., was first involved with what toxicological issue?

He helped *Alzheimer's* patient Janet Adkins end her life with his *"suicide machine."*

❍   In the year 1903, in the town of Enid, Oklahoma, a man named John St. Helens committed suicide by drinking a glass of wine laced with the poison strychnine. This man had claimed that his real identity was that of what notorious individual associated with a famous homicide of the 19th century?

John Wilkes Booth, assassin of President Abraham Lincoln (1865).

❍   In 1834, Hort became the first American physician to use what now commonly used substance, when he saved the life of a patient who had been exposed to Mercuric chloride?

Activated charcoal.

❍   In 1830, the French pharmacist P. F. Touery, was so convinced of the efficacy of Activated charcoal, that in front of his friends, he mixed 15 *grams* of Activated charcoal with several times the lethal dose of a poison, and swallowed the mixture. What poison was he thus able to survive?

Strychnine.

❍   The murder of Gustave Fougnies in 1850, by the Count and Countess de Bocarme, is still the principle example we have of murder by what poison?

Nicotine.

❍   Here are three clues to the identity of a famous toxicologist: FIRST CLUE: Living from 1787-1853, this Spanish physician held a position of respect as attending physician to Louis *XVIII* of France and occupied a chair at the University of Paris. SECOND CLUE: He is often cited as the founder of toxicology by singling out toxicology as a discipline distinct from others, and defined toxicology as the study of poison. THIRD CLUE: In 1814, he published the first general textbook in toxicology, titled *Traite des poisons*. Who was he?

Mattieu Joseph Bonaventura Orfila.

O   Here are three clues to the identity of a famous toxicologist. FIRST CLUE: He was disliked by his peers but was extremely popular with his students and patients, among whom were counted members of many of the ruling families of medieval Europe. SECOND CLUE: Born in 1493, he died in 1541, at the age of 48, as a result of wounds suffered in a tavern brawl in Salzburg. THIRD CLUE: He promoted the view of the *"toxicon,"* the toxic agent, as a chemical entity, and one of his most famous statements was *"Dosis sola facit venenum"* ("The dose alone makes the poison"). Who was he?

Philippus Aureolus Theophrastus Bombastus von Hohenheim-Paracelsus.

O   Members of the nobility have always been targets for poisoners. Therefore, they have gone to great lengths to fight them. Tell whether each of the following persons would wear a white hat (*"good guy"*), or black hat *("bad guy")*: (a) Emperor Shen Nung, (b) King Mitradates *VI*, (c) Catherine de Medici, (d) Marchioness de Brinvilles, (e) Baron Guillaume Dupuytren.

(a) *White* - wrote antidote treatise, (b) *White* - developed universal antidote, (c) *Black* - poisoner, (d) *Black* - poisoner, (e) *White* - early lavage advocate.

O   During history some individuals have been given nicknames which included the word *poison*. Identify the given name of the following individuals: (a) He was called *"Poison Ivy"* by the striking miners of Colorado, for his misrepresentations of the Ludlow strike of 1913-14, (b) This 19th Century murderess estimated to have claimed 31 victims, was called *"Queen Poisoner"* and *"The Modern Lucretia Borgia,"* (c) Teamster Union President Jimmy Hoffa, referred to this government official as *"Poison Snake,"* (d) The son-in-law of Benito Mussolini who tried to keep Italy out of World War II, was referred to as *"That Poisoned Mushroom,"* by Nazi propaganda minister Joseph Goebbels.

(a) Ivy L. Lee (1877-1934), press agent for John D. Rockefeller, (b) Lydia Struck, (c) Robert F. Kennedy, Attorney General, (d) Count Galeazzo Ciano (1903-1944).

O   Some individuals in history have died from poisoning. By what agent did each of the following supposedly meet their end: (a) Cleopatra, (b) Hermann Goering, (c) Emile Zola, (d) Marilyn Monroe.

(a) Asp venom, (b) Cyanide, (c) Carbon monoxide, (d) Barbiturates.

O   Arrange the following famous toxicologists in the correct chronological order when, they made their significant work, from earliest to most current: Orfila, Marsh, Nicander of Colophon, and Thienes.

Nicander of Colophon (200 B.C.), Orfila (1814), Marsh (1836), and Thienes (1900s).

O   Many persons have worked with poisons, some for good and some for evil. Tell whether each of the following persons would wear a white hat (*"good guy"*), or black hat (*"bad guy"*): (a) Donald Harvey, (b) Dr. K.K. Chen, (c) Joseph Orfila, (d) James Marsh, (e) Dr. E.W. Pritchard, (f) Dr. Arthur W. Waite.

(a) *Black* - Nurses Aid Killer, (b) *White* - developed the Cyanide Antidote Kit, (c) *White* – authored toxicology text, (d) *White* - developed Arsenic test, (e) *Black* - murderer by poisons, (f) *Black* - murderer by poisons.

○   Many famous people in history have taken their own lives, some with poison and some by other methods. Indicate whether each of the following committed suicide with poison or by other means: (a) Adolf Hitler, (b) Hannibal, (c) Nero, (d) Judy Garland, (e) Vincent Van Gogh, (f) Ernest Hemingway.

(a) Other - gunshot, (b) Poison, (c) Other - cut throat, (d) Poison - drug overdose, (e) Other -gun shot, (f) Other – gun shot.

○   In 1978, a Bulgarian defector named Georgi Markov, is thought to have been assassinated in a rather unique manner when a hollow metal sphere containing poison was implanted under his skin by an unknown assailant. Answer the following about this incident: (a) In what European city did this incident occur, (b) What was the implement thought to be used to deliver the sphere, (c) What toxin was the sphere supposed to have contained?

(a) London, England, (b) An umbrella, (c) Ricin, the phytotoxin from *Ricinus communus*, Castor Bean.

○   Here are three clues to the identity of an infamous poisoner. FIRST CLUE: An American born physician, this individual moved to England in 1900, where the spouse was subsequently murdered utilizing hyoscine. SECOND CLUE: This individual was captured trying to flee by ship, by the first utilization of the new Marconi "wireless" radio, in the apprehension of a criminal. THIRD CLUE: This man's name has become synonymous with POISONER and has earned him a place in the *"Chamber of Horrors,"* of *Madame Tussad's Wax Museum* in London, England. Who was this person?

Hawley Harvey Crippen, M.D. (1862-1910).

○   Many persons have worked with poisons, some for good and some for evil. Tell whether each of the following persons would wear a white hat (*"good guy"*), or black hat (*"bad guy"*): (a) Ronald Clark O'Bryan, (b) Graham Young, (c) Sadamichi Hirasaywa, (d) Henry Parrish, (e) Hugo Reinsch, (f) Henri Girard.

(a) *Black* - The Candy Man, (b) *Black* - poisoner, (c) *Black* - Cyanide bank robber, (d) *White*-snake bite epidemiologist, (e) *White* - developed test for arsenic, (f) *Black* - the first "scientific" poisoner.

○   Here are three clues to the identity of a famous scientific individual who possibly suffered a toxicological malady. FIRST CLUE: He was born on December 25, 1642, and by the time he was 50 years of age (1692), he had begun to suffer from a form of mental "madness" that ended his scientific career. SECOND CLUE: It has been argued that his mental problems arose from the metals mercury and lead, which had entered his system during his many experiments in the area of Alchemy.

THIRD CLUE: He died on March 20, 1727, but the world has a much better understanding of gravitational forces because of his work. Who was he?

Sir Isaac Newton.

❍   **What toxicologist's name(s) is/are associated with the following nomograms: (a) Acetaminophen toxicity, (b) Salicylate toxicity.**

(a) Rumack-Matthew, (b) Done.

❍   **In 1990, Paul Stedman Cullen Jr., was convicted of a most unusual intentional poisoning. Answer the following about this incident: (a) What was the name of the poison that was used, (b) In what city did this incident take place, (c) Who, or what, was the victim of this crime.**

(a) The herbicide Velpar, (b) Austin, Texas, (c) A tree, the historic *"Treaty Oak,"* which was estimated to be 500 years old.

❍   **This English homicidal poisoner, who began experimenting with poisons on the members of his own family, is one of the primary examples of a *"toxicomaniac"* in the history of homicidal poisoning. He eventually died in a British prison in 1989. Who was he?**

Graham Frederick Young.

❍   **This famous British toxicologist worked under Orfila in Paris, went on to be professor of medical jurisprudence at the University of Edinburgh, and was called as a toxicological expert at the famous 1857 trial of Madeleine Smith. Who was he?**

Robert Christison (1797-1882).

❍   **In 1775, the British physician William Withering discovered the therapeutic effects on *"dropsy"* (Congestive Heart Failure) of the toxic plant *Digitalis*. At the time he was the physician of what famous visiting American diplomat?**

Benjamin Franklin.

❍   **The first murderer to be arrested through the use of a telegram, when a description of him was sent to the British police in 1845, was a poisoner. Who was he?**

John Tawell.

❍   **This talented artist wanted to be an entomologist, but was afraid of taking physics. Instead, he used his talents as a cartoonist to create some of the most humorous renditions involving animals, many of which are toxic. What is the name of this very popular naturalist-theme cartoonist?**

Gary Larson.

❍   In 1957, the famed zoologist Karl Schmidt, of the *Field Museum of Natural History* in Chicago, Illinois, died the next day after being bitten by what type of African venomous snake he was handling to study?

A "Boomslang."

❍   What American President of the 1800s believed so strongly in the antidotal power of a *"madstone"* that he took his son Robert to the possessor of such an item when he had been bitten by a snake?

Abraham Lincoln.

❍   A biography of this famous Italian artist/scientist, by the Russian writer Marezhovski, stated that he had used cyanide to commit the perfect crime. Who was this respected man?

Leonardo da Vinci.

❍   *"I feel sick. My head is splitting. No, don't you see the dog is sick too. We are both ill. It must be something we have eaten. It will pass away. Let us not bother them."* On September 28, 1902, these were the final words of what French writer, who was to succumb to the effects of carbon monoxide poisoning from a faulty stove in his Paris apartment?

Emile Zola, as said to his wife.

❍   In 1972, the photographer W. Eugene Smith, won the *Pulitzer Prize* for his famous photograph showing the effects of *"Minamata Disease"* on a patient. What was the title of this award winning photo?

"Tomoko in Bath."

❍   Sometimes people who are very hungry will even eat spoiled food, paying no attention to the potential for food poisoning. What Asian world leader once said: *"To a man with an empty stomach, food is God."*?

Mohandas K. Gandi.

❍   This scientist, who lived from 1813-1878, first identified the site of action of the poison Curare. He stated *"the physiological analysis of organic systems...can be done with the aid of toxic agents."* Who was he?

Claude Bernard.

❍   This Belgian chemist, who lived from 1813-1891, developed a method of extracting alkaloids from cadavers, which became the first effective method of extraction of organic poisons from biological materials. Who was he?

Jean Servais Stas.

❍   What jazz performer in 1933, sang a song, with the lyrics: *"Cocaine for horses an' not for men, doctors say it'll kill you, but they don't say when. An' ho, ho, baby, take a whiff on me."* Who was this personage?

Leadbelly, in the song *"Take a Whiff on Me."*

❍   In the mid 1970s, an enterprising truck driver named Edward Seay, began merchandising what products from the *Seay Drug Company* of Union City, Georgia, that caused a great deal of confusion with the toxicologic community?

OTC stimulant drugs made to look like *Schedule III* and *IV* amphetamines and stimulants, or *"turkey drugs."*

❍   In the late 1800s, the famous sexologist Havelock Ellis dabbled with what hallucinogenic substance, and described many benefits from its use?

Mescaline.

❍   An 18th century ship's doctor named Thomas Dover became famous for the creation of *"Dover's Powders,"* a powdered opium formulation, which lead to many addictions. But he is also famous for his rescue of a remotely stranded traveler. Who was this fortunate nautical traveler?

Alexander Selkirk, *aka "Robinson Crusoe."*

❍   This famous American zoo director, although severely envenomated by the bite of a Gaboon Viper (*Biti gabonica*), survived and went on to become a television personality, bringing the natural world into the home of the viewing audience. Who was he?

Marlin Perkins.

❍   In the 1990s, Qiu Mantan, China's self-proclaimed *"King of Rat Killers,"* invented a commercial rat poison containing a prohibited ingredient. What was the ingredient?

Fluoroacetamide, Compound *"1081."*

❍   What physician is credited with the first description of abdominal colic, in a patient who was a metal extractor?

Hippocrates (370 BC).

❍   According to the magazine *High Times,* what Hungarian celebrity admitted on "The Maury Povich Show" to smoking marijuana with a horse?

Zsa Zsa Gabor.

❍   **Edward Press and Louis Gdalman were the co-founders of the first poison center in the USA. What profession were these two individuals practicing when this important event took place?**

They were both pharmacists.

❍   **Dr. Theodore Morell (1887-1948), was a morphine addict, but he had a famous patient into whom he injected drugs laced with atropine and strychnine. Who was his famous European patient?**

Adolf Hitler (1889-1945).

❍   **Richard Barter (1834-1859), a California robber, was known by what nickname that was associated with a toxic critter?**

"Rattlesnake Dick."

❍   **On August 26, 1978, this French born screen actor, known for his roles as a romantic lover, committed suicide by taking an overdose of barbiturates. Who was he?**

Chalres Boyer (1899-1978).

❍   **On March 13, 1990, this famous U.S. psychologist, a pioneer in autism and other *"problem"* children, committed suicide by means of barbiturates and smothering with a plastic bag. Who was he?**

Bruno Bettelheim (1903-1990).

❍   **On May 2, 1945, this high ranking Nazi figure, attempting to flee from Berlin, and trapped by cross-fire near the *Lehrter* railroad station, supposedly ended his life by swallowing cyanide. What was his name?**

Martin Bormann (1900-1945).

❍   **On March 1, 1983, this Hungarian author of *Darkness at Noon*, committed suicide along with his wife, by taking an overdose of Tuinal® (secobarbital + amobarbital). His suicide was probably due to the fact he could not face his terminal cancer. Who was this author?**

Arthur Koestler (1905-1983).

❍   **On January 29, 1933, this famous lady poet of America, committed suicide with a heavy dose of sleeping pills.   She had won the *Pulitzer Prize* in 1917, for her *Love Songs*. Who was this famous literary woman?**

Sara Teasdale (1884-1933).

❍   Around June 8, 1954, this famous English mathematician apparently committed suicide by eating an apple which had been dipped in potassium cyanide. His early works lead to the concept of the electronic computer. Who was he?

Alan M. Turing (1912-1954).

❍   In the 1850s, the famous Lola Montez, entertained the miners and residents of the California gold rush, with a famous dance, which was named the same as a toxic critter. What was the name of the dance?

The *"Spider Dance."*

❍   What explorer, while alone in 1934, at an isolated outpost in Antarctica, became extremely ill when he was so overcome by fumes from a generator, that he had to be rescued by a team of his fellow researchers.

Admiral Richard E. Byrd.

❍   Charlie Brooks Jr., had a toxic encounter on December 7, 1982, in Huntsville, Texas. What made this an historic first?

He was the first American murderer executed by lethal injection.

❍   The artists Manet, Degas, Van Gogh, and Picasso all created artwork which depicted a toxic substance. What was the substance so depicted?

The use of the popular, and toxic drink, *"absinthe."*

❍   What famous English explorer wrote the following in 1595: *"There was nothing where of I was more curious than to find out the true remedies of these poisoned arrows. For besides the mortality of the wounds they make, the party shot endureth the most insufferable torment in the world and abideth a most ugly and lamentable death."*?

Sir Walter Raleigh.

❍   On December 17, 1947, Sir Bernard Spillsbury, one of the most prominent forensic pathologists of Great Britain, ended his long career, by committing suicide in his laboratory. What method did he use?

Natural gas asphyxiation.

❍   This Italian physician was the first to describe the venom apparatus of snakes in his 1664 book *De Venenis Animalibus*. Who was this pioneer researcher?

Francesco Redi (1626-1697).

❍   What Philadelphia neurologist, published a significant study on rattlesnake venom in 1860, titled *Researches Upon the Venom of the Rattlesnake*?

Silas Wier Mitchell (1829-1914).

O   **According to a popular children's rhyme of the period, fill in the blank with the name of the infamous female poisoner is being alluded to:** *"Mary Ann [blank], She's dead and rotten. She lies in her bed, With her eyes wide open."*

Cotton (1832-1873).

O   **In the 1920s, the chef of the *"Little Italy Cafe,"* who eventually chickened out, was offered $10,000 to put Cyanide in the soup of what prominent underworld leader?**

Alphonse Capone.

O   **In 1917, there was an abortive assassination attempt on the life of a British Prime Minister, by utilizing an air gun with Curare tipped darts. Who was their intended target?**

Lloyd George.

O   **This famous British military leader and founder of the empire of British India, who lived from 1725-1774, became addicted to Opium. Who was he?**

Robert Clive.

O   **In 1943, Dr. Albert Hoffman had a toxicological vision. What was the cause of this phenomenon?**

The accidental discoverer of *LSD*, he experimentally took 40 *mcg*.

O   **This 16th Century diplomat introduced tobacco into France. The major toxic constituent Nicotine was named in his honor. What was his name?**

Jean Nicot.

O   **What actress, found dead on July 1, 1996, of a Phenobarbital overdose, followed in the footsteps of her famous grandfather, who also committed suicide?**

Margeaux Hemingway.

O   **The Dutch physician Hermann Boerhaave is given the honor of being the first to suggest a chemical method of proving the presence of poisons. What was his method?**

He stated that various poisons in a *"red hot or vaporous condition"* yielded various typical odors.

O   **Although initially thought to be guilty, in 1984, what automotive wonder kid was acquitted for dealing in the sale of Cocaine?**

John DeLorean.

O   **Who was the first American physician to devote their career to the practice of industrial medicine, and who in 1925 wrote the groundbreaking book *Industrial Poisons in the United States*?**

Dr. Alice Hamilton (1869-1970).

O   **The great Greek tragedian Euripides (480-406 BC), in a single day, lost his wife and three children from exposure to what toxic entity?**

Mushrooms.

O   **What Czech musician, composer of the *"New World Symphony,"* lost his 10 month old daughter in 1877, after she ate phosphorus?**

Anton Dvorak.

O   **What notorious female poisoner of Naples, Italy, executed in 1723, was later used as the protagonist in *"Sidonia the Sorceress"*?**

Madame La Toffana.

O   **The April 3, 1995 issue of *Time* magazine declared what individual the *"Prophet of Poison"*?**

Shoko Asahara, founder of the *Aum Shinrikyo* cult.

O   **She was born in 1876, in the Netherlands, as Margaret Gertrude Zelle. Around 1900, in Java, her young son was homicidally poisoned by an irate housekeeper. She returned to Europe as an exotic dancer, and in 1917, was shot by the French as a spy. By what more exotic name was she known?**

Mata Hari.

O   **In 1761, Sir John Hill first associated the excessive use of what substance with its carcinogenic potential, causing malignant nasal polyps?**

Snuff.

O   **What great Victorian explorer was the first to describe the native use of species of *Strophanthus* for arrow poisons?**

Dr. David Livingstone.

O   **When he was 19 years old, his mother killed herself by drinking hydrochloric acid. In later life his espionage activities gave away the details of one of America's great secrets. On what activity was spy Klaus Fuchs privy to details?**

The *"Manhattan Project,"* the making of the atomic bomb.

O   In 1767, the gifted composer and organist at the court of Versailles, Johann Scholert, died along with his wife and most of his children from exposure to what toxic entity?

Mushrooms.

O   In the year 1812, at the *Chateau de Fontainebleau*, this European political leader unsuccessfully attempted suicide with poison.   Who was this dynamic individual?

Napoleon Bonaparte.

O   In Paris in 1938, Lev Sedev was presumably poisoned by a Russian agent. Lev was the son of what famous Russian revolutionary who had fallen out of favor with the other leaders?

Leon Trotsky.

O   Chemist Fritz Haber eventually went on to win a Nobel Prize. But, for his work in his earlier career, he could be considered the *"father"* of what toxic mode combat weapon?

Chemical Warfare.

O   In late March, 1997, a mass suicide of 39 cult members took place in the U.S.A., utilizing poison as their tool. Answer the following about this horrific event: (a) Where did this suicide occur, (b) What was the name of the cult, (c) What was the name of the cult's leader, (d) What two substances were used as suicidal agents, (e) What was the goal of the members that brought about this action?

(a) Rancho Sante Fe, California, (b) *"Heaven's Gate,"* (c) Marshall Applewhite, aka *"Do,"* (d) phenobarbital in applesauce consumed with vodka, (e) they wanted to join with a UFO behind the *"Hale-Bopp"* comet.

O   Here are clues to the identity of a popular personage. FIRST CLUE: I am a TV actress whose younger sister died from combining dextropoxyphene with ethanol. SECOND CLUE: I tried to help my brother overdose on morphine and analgesics when he was dying from cancer. THIRD CLUE: My name could come to mind when people talk of the infamous poisoner, Blanche Taylor Moore.

Mary Tyler Moore.

O   Arrange the following personages in toxicology in chronological order from most ancient to most recent: Peter Abbonus, Shen Nung, Francis Megende, Richard Mead.

Sheng Nung (~2,000 BC) > Peter Abbonus (1250-1315) > Richard Mead (1673-1754) > Francis Megende (1783-1855).

○   **In 1812, Physick used what new method to treat two infants who had been overdosed on laudanum?**

Lavage.

○   **In September 1954, an Australian named Kirke Dyson-Holland died from a venomous bite. This was the first recorded case of a fatality from what marine animal?**

"Blue-ringed Octopus."

○   **In World War II, this U.S. dancer was slated for murder by the Gestapo for marrying a Jewish businessman. Goering invited her to dinner with plans of putting cyanide in her fish course. Because she was forewarned she was able to avoid a violent death. Living from 1906-1975, she stormed Paris in the 1920s, and was the first black woman to appear in the *"Folies-Begeriere."* Who was she?**

Josephine Baker.

○   **When he was a small boy, this future famous 18th century American writer and diplomat said to his mother *"I have imbibed an acephalous molluscosus,"* upon which his mother thinking he had eaten a poison gave him a large dose of an emetic. After he told her it was nothing but an oyster, she thrashed him for deceiving her. After that he said he would never use big words, when little ones would do. Who was this famous American patriot?**

Benjamin Franklin.

○   **The first lawsuit won by a black against a white man in the United States occurred in 1836, when a black domestic servant won a slander suit again the man who had accused her of poisoning with arsenic laced coffee. The woman who won the suit late became a famous women's rights activist, visited Abraham Lincoln, and made more famous by her *"Ain't I A Woman?"* speech. Who was she?**

Sojourner Truth (*aka* Isabella Van Wagemen).

○   **For a long time it was believed he died of mercury or lead poisoning, but in 1999 analysis of his hair ruled out toxic levels of these metals. Answer the following about this American President: (a) What was his name, (b) What numbered President was he?**

(a) Andrew Jackson, (b) 7th.

○   **Born in 1922, I was the first black actress to make it big in Hollywood, and the first African-American to be nominated for an *Academy Award* for best actress. I died in 1965, from an overdose of Amitriptyline, although it was never determined whether it was accidental or suicidal. Who was I?**

Dorothy Dandridge.

❍   **Who once said** *"I think that I had better bathe before I drink the poison, and not give the women the trouble of washing my dead body"*?

Socrates (as quoted in Plato's *Phaedio*).

❍   **What famous choreographer once said** *"Most ballet dancers in the United States are terrible. If they were in medicine, everyone would be poisoned."*?

George Balanchine (1904-1983).

❍   **What United States college football coach once said** *"Publicity is like poison; it doesn't hurt unless you swallow it"*?

Joe Paterno.

❍   **What popular flat affect comedian said** *"My girlfriend and I went on a picnic. I don't know how she did it, but she got poison ivy on the brain. When it itched, the only way she could scratch it was to think about sandpaper."*?

Steven Wright.

❍   **In 1856, what infamous poisoner about to be executed, surprisingly said to the executioner as he stepped onto the shaky trap of the gallows,** *"Are you sure it's safe?"*

William Palmer, MD (1824-1856).

❍   **In 2000, Monica Traub was fired as the kitchen maid to what royal personage after supposedly making statements about how easy it would be to poison this person with cyanide?**

Queen Elizabeth *II*, of the United Kingdom.

❍   **Raphael de Rothschild, scion of the famed banking family, died on April 22, 2000 on a Chelsea sidewalk from exposure to what toxic substance?**

Heroin.

❍   **Captain John Smith (of Pocahantas fame) was once accused of poisoning Dutch settlers with** *Ratsbane*. **What is** *Ratsbane*?

Arsenic trioxide.

❍   **Give the first four given names of the famous alchemist-toxicologist known as Paracelsus.**

Phillipus, Aureolus, Theophrastus, Bombastus.

❍   **Who was the counsel for the Chairman of the** *Philip Morris Company* **during the 1993 Congressional hearings on tobacco and health?**

Kenneth Starr (of Clinton scandal fame).

○   **On August 17, 1962, President Kennedy awarded a medal to what physician who was instrumental for her role in the prevention of the *thalidomide* disaster in the United States?**

Dr. Frances Kelsey.

PLANTS AND FUNGI

○ **Which of the following plants does NOT cause cardiac toxicity:** *Foxglove, Lily-of-the-Valley, Mountain Laurel, Mayapple,* **or** *Oleander?*

Mayapple.

○ **At Christmas time we find this plant part used in a popular drink, but in the prison population it has been abused as a hallucinogenic. What is the common name of this plant material?**

Nutmeg, the fruit of the tree *Myristica fragrans.*

○ **To the careful ear, the names of various plants may sound like other things. What plant, which can cause dermatitis like poison ivy, has an edible nut, and whose name sounds like a sneeze?**

Cashew.

○ **One of the first prominent Americans to eat a berry which was considered poisonous (but now accepted as edible), was Thomas Jefferson. What is the more common name of this fruit?**

The tomato.

○ **What plant was: cultivated by the Aztecs, referred to by the Mexicans as** *flores de noche buena* **("flowers of the Holy Night"), and is often involved in holiday exposures?**

Poinsettia.

○ **In 1986, the National Flower of the United States of America was designated. Is it from a toxic plant?**

No, it is the rose.

○ *Tremetol* **poisoning is contracted by humans who drink milk from cows which have consumed "Snakeroot" (***Eupatorium rugosum***). This poisoning is thought to have taken the lives of the mother, great-aunt, great-uncle, and second cousin of what 19th century American President?**

Abraham Lincoln.

❍   The Canadian flag features the red maple leaf. To what non-human animal has the red maple been shown to be toxic?

The horse.

❍   According to mythology, what poisonous plant was created by *Hecate* (goddess of the underworld) from the saliva of *Cerberus* (the three-headed dog that guarded the gates of *Hades*)?

"Monkshood," *Aconitum napellus*.

❍   According to mythology, what poisonous plant "formed the cup" that *Medea* prepared for *Theseus*.

"Monkshood," *Aconitum napellus*.

❍   Why is the poisonous plant *"Monkshood"* sometimes referred to as *"Wolfsbane"*?

Because arrows dipped in the poison could be used to kill wolves.

❍   These resinoid plants toxins are found in the honey, nectar, leaves, and flowers, of many of the genera (such as *Kalmia*, *Pieris*, and *Rhododendron*) of family Ericaceae. As a group, what are these toxins called?

Grayanotoxins.

❍   Concern about poisonous plants was so great that this group of early 19th century American explorers only purchased wild plants from Indians who regularly ate the plants as foods. What was the name of the famous expedition?

The Lewis and Clark Expedition.

❍   Growing in field bottoms, the plant *Crotalaria sagittalis*, known as the *"Rattlebox,"* is thought to have caused what named disease state which resulted in the deaths of horses in the 1800s?

"Bottom Disease."

❍   In 1830, on Vancouver Island, Canada, David Douglas is given credit for discovering *"Western Poison Oak."* What common nontoxic plant is named after this famed British botanist?

Douglas Fir.

❍   This German was the first toxicologist to study psychoactive plants and, in 1924 published *Phantastica*, which examined 28 plants used around the world for their stimulating effects. What was the name of this toxicologist?

Louis Lewin.

❍   One of the oldest plants known to be poisonous, it is also known as *Bois joli*, *Dwarf Bay*, *Wood laurel*, and *Flax olive*. But what is the common name?

Daphne.

❍   The term *"dwale,"* popular in the time of Chaucer, and meaning *"to sleep,"* was applied to what toxic plant?

"Deadly nightshade."

❍   What native Hawaiian dish is prepared from the oxalate containing Taro plant?

"Poi."

❍   This toxic plant gets its name from the Greek word *"athanasia"* for "immortality." It was the main ingredient in a potion supposedly given to *Ganymede*, who became a cupbearer for *Zeus*. It may have gotten its name from the fact its flowers do not wilt easily, and was often placed in coffins as in insect repellent. What is the more common name of this plant?

Tansy, *Tanacetum vulgare.*

❍   This common toxic plant is found all over the world and has many common names. In China, it is called *"tan chi,"* in Japan *"tsuta urushi."* To French Canadians it is *"herbe a la puce"* or *"herb of the flea."* By what common name do most Americans call this plant?

"Poison Ivy."

❍   The first European to describe Poison Ivy was remembered more for his liaison with Pocohontas. Who was he?

Captain John Smith.

❍   The shield of Quebec and Ontario display the leaves of a plant. Is it considered a poisonous plant to humans?

No, it is the maple leaf.

❍   This toxic plant containing anticholinergic alkaloids was associated with a mass exposure near Jamestown, Virginia during *Bacon's Rebellion* in 1676. What is the scientific name of the plant which became known as *"Jimson Weed"* because of this incident?

Datura stramonium.

❍   What toxic plant is the State Flower of West Virginia and Washington?

Rhododendron.

❍   The *FDA* noted that there may be a problem with certain brands of cheap vanilla extract being sold south of the border. What plant used to adulterate the vanilla, and possibly leading to coagulation alterations, is the problem?

"Tonka Bean."

❍   Having killed up to 13 of 18 victims, as early as the first 7 hours after ingestion (in 1934 and 1937), the mushroom *Galerina sulcipes* is thought to be the world's most toxic. On what Asian island did these most disastrous deaths occur?

Java, Indonesia.

❍   The very toxic seed of the plant *Abrus precatorius*, also known as the *"Rosary Pea"* or *"Doll's Eye,"* grows in a pod, like a pea. On which end of the seed, red or black, is the seed attachment?

The black end.

❍   Certain species of this genus of mushroom contain cyclopeptides which can be very toxic to the kidneys. This genus which is NOT *Amanita*, is genus what?

Cortinarius, which contain Orelline and Orellanine.

❍   *"Red squill"* is a plant product that is best utilized to combat what group of pests?

Rodents.

❍   What species of plant, considered one of the most toxic in the world, has a brilliantly colored red and black seed?

Abrus precatorius, "Rosary Pea," "Doll's Eyes."

❍   What is the name of the mushroom which causes an Antabuse-like reaction when consumed with ethanol?

"Inky-Cap," or *Coprinus atramentarius*.

❍   A quick field test for the presence of amatoxins in mushroom tissue consists of spotting tissue juice on newsprint and adding a drop of concentrated hydrochloric acid. What is the more common name for this test?

"Meixner Test" (more correctly called the *"Wieland Test"*).

❍   What is the name of the only church in the U.S. that has been sanctioned to use *Peyote* in its religious ceremonies?

Native American Church.

❍   The Germans called it *"fingerhut,"* to the French it was known as *"gentelee."* In Ireland it was called the *"fairy cup"* and in Wales it was known as *"goblin's gloves."* In some parts of England it was known as *"witches' bells"* or *"fairy folks glove."* Its common name comes from *"digitale"* (a thimble or finger stall). What is the genus name of this toxic plant?

Digitalis.

❍   What plant alkaloid was worth $2,200 per ounce in 1981?

Cocaine.

❍   In Norse mythology, the god *Baldur* was killed by a dart made from a poisonous plant. What was the name of the plant used?

"Mistletoe," *Viscum album.*

❍   Perhaps the most famous cookbook in the world, *Larousse Gastronomique,* once erroneously declared that the toxic leaves of what plant could be *"eaten like spinach"*?

Rhubarb, *Rheum rhaponticum.*

❍   In the 1960's, members of the drug culture bought packages of seeds of varieties such as *"Flying Saucers," "Pearly Gates," "Blue Stars," "Summer Skies,"* and *"Wedding Bells,"* in order to consume them to get a psychoactive experience. What is the common name of the plant which these varieties represented?

Morning Glories, species of genus *Ipomoea,* which contained *LSD*-like compounds.

❍   What fruit, often mistaken for a vegetable, did American colonists call a *"Love Apple"* and avoid believing it to be poisonous?

The tomato, *Lycopersicon esculentum.*

❍   In 1969, a group of French soldiers on a survival course, all died after eating what genus of plant which they had cooked thinking it was edible?

Aconitum.

❍   Prussia's Frederick William *I,* passed a law stating that anyone who did NOT grow this member of the *Solanum* genus, would have their ears and nose cut off! What is the name of this plant?

The potato, *Solanum tuberosum.*

❍   Each of the following plants contain a very toxic compound commonly called a *toxalbumin* or *phytotoxin.* Name the compound found in each of the following plants: (a) Castor Bean, (b) Black Locust, (c) Rosary Peas.

(a) *Ricin*, (b) *Robin*, (c) *Abrin.*

❍   **Tell whether the berries of the following plants are considered toxic or nontoxic: (a) *Phorodendron serotinum*, (b) *Rubus ideaus*, (c) *Celastrus scandens*, (d) *Menispermum canidense*, (e) *Sorbus ancuparia.***

(a) Toxic, *"Mistletoe,"* (b) Non-toxic, *"Red Raspberry,"* (c) Toxic, *"Bittersweet,"* (d) Toxic, "Moonseed," (e) Non-toxic, *"Mountain Ash."*

❍   **Give the common name for each of the following toxic plants: (a) *Convallaria majalis*, (b) *Cicuta maculata*, (c) *Abrus precatorius*, (d) *Conium maculatum*, (e) *Phytolacca americana.***

(a) *"Lilly-of-the-Valley,"* (b) *"Water hemlock,"* (c) *"Rosary Pea,"* or *"Doll's Eye,"* (d) *"Poison Hemlock,"* (e) *"Pokeweed,"* or *"Inkberry."*

❍   **The names of many poisonous plants have interesting origins. Identify, by common or scientific name, each of the following plants from the descriptions of their name origin. (a) Its genus name derives from the Latin for *"comforting"* and the species name (part Greek and part Latin) means false-pepper; (b) Its berries being quite attractive to children, this plant's common name comes from the Algonquian Indian word *"puccoon"* (a plant used for staining or dying); (c) Being immediately painful upon contact, this plant's genus name is the original Latin name for the plant, while the species name comes from the Greek for *"two households"* indicating that the male and female flowers are usually found on separate plants; (d) This plant's genus name comes from the Latin for *"tick"* which its seed resembles. The species name comes from the Latin for *"growing in communities,"* indicating its gregarious growth habit; (e) The common name of this ornamental houseplant was given in memory of the first ambassador to Mexico from the U.S., who later introduced this plant to South Carolina; (f) The common garden plant derives its genus name from Latin word for a *"valley,"* a reference to the favored habitat. The species name means *"flowering in May."***

(a) *Solanum pseudocapsicum*, or "Jerusalem Cherry," (b) "Pokeweed," or *Phytolacca americana*, (c) *Urtica dioica*, or "Stinging Nettle," (d) *Ricinus communis*, or "Castor-oil Plant," (e) "Poinsettia" (for Joel R. Poinsette 1775-1851), or *Euphorbia pulcherrima*, (f) *Convallaria majalis*, or "Lilly-of-the-Valley."

❍   **Are you able to tell one hemlock from another? Give the genus or common name for the plant being described: (a) This hemlock can cause convulsions and resembles a plant known as *"Wild Carrot,"* (b) This hemlock causes muscle weakness and paralysis, its seeds resemble anise seeds, and smell like mouse urine, (c) This hemlock is actually a conifer tree, and is NOT toxic.**

(a) *Cicuta*, also known as "Water Hemlock," (b) *Conium*, also known as "Poison Hemlock," (c) *Tsuga*, also known as "Western Hemlock."

❍   **Many poisonous plants have the word *"bane"* in their common name. Given the scientific name, provide for each, the *"baneful"* common name: (a) *Aconitum*** *napellus*, (b) *Hyoscyamus niger*, (c) *Cicuta virosa*, (d) *Apocynum androsaemifolium*, (e) *Actaea alba*.

(a) "Wolfsbane," (b) "Henbane," (c) "Cowbane," (d) "Dogbane," (e) "White baneberry."

○ **What are the five macroscopic characteristics which identify the "Fly Agaric" mushroom, *Amanita muscaria*?**

(a) *Vulva*, or "death cup," (b) *Annulus*, or "skirt," (c) White gills, or free gills, (d) Patches on the cap surface, (e) Orange to red color of the cap surface.

○ **For each of the following mushroom species, indicate whether one would expect anticholinergic, cholinergic, or neither symptoms, from their intoxication: (a) *Coprinus atramentarius*, (b) *Amanita pantherina*, (c) *Gyromitra esculenta*, (d) *Amanita muscaria*, (e) *Clitocybe dealbata*.**

(a) Neither, (b) Anticholinergic, (c) Neither, (d) Anticholinergic, (e) Cholinergic.

○ **In the West Indies, ingestion of the immature *aril* of this tropical evergreen causes a condition known as *"Jamaican Vomiting Sickness."* Answer the following about this plant: (a) What is the common name of this plant, and (b) What infamous naval captain was the genus of this plant named in honor of?**

(a) *"Akee,"* (b) Captain William (*"Bounty"*) Bligh, *Blighia sapida*.

○ **One may mow over these mushrooms in one's yard, but don't pick them up and put them in one's pocket, as one will be subject to arrest. What group of mushrooms are considered illegal to possess?**

Those containing psychoactive substances, which are considered a *"Schedule I"* controlled substance (*e.g. Psilocybe spp., Panaeolus spp., Gymnopilus spp., etc.*).

○ **Many species of this genus of plants are toxic, and the genus was named in honor of a physician to Juba, King of Mauritania. What is the name of this plant genus?**

Euphorbia, named for *Euphorbus*.

○ **This plant has very toxic seeds. The genus comes from the Greek for *"delicate,"* and the species from *"entreating."* What is the scientific name of this plant?**

Abrus precatorius.

○ **This plant genus is named after a province in Asia Minor, where the hardy bulb plant abounds. What is the name of the genus?**

Colchicum, after the province of Colchis.

❍   The genus of this plant is named for one of the *"Three Fates"* of Grecian mythology, from whom there was no escape, alluding to the poisonous berries. What is the genus of these toxic plants?

Atropa, named after *Atropos*.

❍   This plant genus, which contains members with painful effects when chewed, is named in honor of a German botanist. What is the plant genus?

Dieffenbachia, named in honor of Dr. Dieffenbach.

❍   This toxic plant genus, is named from the Latin name for the tree, and perhaps comes from the Greek word for *"bow,"* as the wood was once used in the making of such weapons. What is the plant genus?

Taxus, the "Yew."

❍   Although the species name of this mushroom, *muscaria*, would lead one to think that the major toxic compound would be *muscarine*, in actuality, there is another more prevalent toxic compound. What is it?

Ibotenic Acid, or *Muscimol*.

❍   When immigrants from Asia come to the United States, they often erroneously collect our very toxic "Death Cap," *Amanita phalloides*, thinking it is the same as an edible species that grows in their homelands. What is the scientific name of the mushroom that is collected and eaten back home?

Amanita princeps.

❍   What is the toxic compound found in the *"Ordeal Bean of Calabar,"* which in the 1800s, was described as being used in *"trial by poison,"* at the mouth of the Niger River, along the Calabar coast of West Africa?

Physostigmine.

❍   The plant known as "Bitter Cassava" (*Manihot esculenta*) contains toxic cyanide compounds. But when properly treated it becomes edible. What is the common Cassava plant product found on sale in most northern supermarkets?

Tapioca.

❍   What is morphologically unusual about the Mexican hallucinogenic plant *Rhyncosia pyramidalis*, that to the uneducated eye makes it look like a another very toxic plant?

It has red and black seeds like the plant *Abrus precatorius*, except the seed attachment is at the red end.

❍   **Most people know that tobacco can be poisonous in large quantities, but what other plant has the common name of *"Poison Tobacco"*?**

"Henbane," *Hyoscyamus niger.*

❍   **Because of its ability to glow in the dark, and its intense orange color, the mushroom *Clitocybe illudens* or *Omphalotus ollearius*, which causes gastrointestinal irritation, is commonly referred to by what common name?**

The *"Jack-o'-Lantern"* mushroom.

❍   **It is known that certain species of the mushroom genus *Amanita* contain very toxic amatoxin cyclopeptides, but two species of the mushroom genus *Lepiota* are also known to contain these compounds. What two species have been associated with human fatalities in North America?**

Lepiota josserandii, and *Lepiota subincarnata.*

❍   **What mushroom toxin's name is derived from the Japanese words for: *"with warts"* + *"long-nosed goblin"* + *"mushroom"*?**

Ibotenic acid, from *"ibo-tengu-take,"* their name for *Amanita strobiliformis.*

❍   **Named for the shape of its flower, this toxic plant's common name is associated with the political intrigue among the ranks of the Roman Catholic clergy. What is the plant?**

"Monkshood," *Aconitum spp.*

❍   **Its hard to believe that rockets and mushrooms have something in common that is toxic. What is it?**

The chemical Monomethylhydrazine (MMH), which is a rocket propellant as well as a toxic compound found in certain species of *Gyromitra*.

❍   **It is said that because the wood of this plant had been used to make the cross of Jesus Christ, that the plant was thereafter forced to exist totally as a parasite. What is the common name of this toxic holiday plant?**

Mistletoe.

❍   **What mushroom toxin's molecular structure is unusual because it contains a cyclopropane ring?**

Coprine.

❍   **What is unusual about the mushroom *Coprinites dominicana*?**

Found encased in amber, it is the oldest known gilled mushroom, at 40 million years.

❍   **In the 1930s, a treatment popular in France for intoxication by the cyclopeptides of the *Amanita* mushrooms, was known as the *"Therapy of Limosen."* What were the fresh ingredients of this supposed antidote?**

The raw brains and stomachs of rabbits.

❍   **In 1869, the first mushroom toxin was isolated. What toxin was it?**

Muscarine.

❍   **A U.S. patent was issued in 1969, to use what mushroom toxin as a flavor enhancer?**

Ibotenic acid.

❍   **What close cousin of the toxic *"Deadly Nightshade"* plant is sold in many fast food restaurants as a popular food for teenagers?**

The "Potato," *Solanum tuberosum.*

❍   **What is the common or scientific name of the plant which gives the breath a characteristic odor of *"Worcestershire"* sauce?**

"Devil's Dung," *Ferula asafoetida.*

❍   **The plant *"Hemlock Water Dropwork"* (*Oenanathe crocata*), has another necro-related common name. What is it?**

"Dead Men's Fingers."

❍   **What poisonous plant's toxic compound gives it the characteristic odor of mouse urine?**

The compound *Coniine* in "Hemlock," *Conium maculatum.*

❍   **What West Indian plant was supposedly used to control slaves by keeping them from talking back to their masters?**

"Dumb Cane," *Dieffenbachia.*

❍   **What nontoxic plant's berries, commonly eaten by children, are usually found growing in pairs on a single pedicel, which makes identification easier?**

"Honeysuckle," *Lonicera spp.*

❍   **Both Pliny the Elder, and Dioscorides, described an insect repellant made from the juice of what toxic plant?**

"Wormwood."

❍   **Count Filip Johan von Strhlenberg, who was a *POW* in Siberia for a many years, reported an unusual practice among Siberians, where people would drink the urine of a person, or reindeer, intoxicated by mushrooms, for hallucinogenic actions. What was the intoxicating mushroom used?**

The "Fly Agaric," *Amanita muscaria.*

❍   **The *"Malay Fish Berry"* contains an alkaloid formerly used to treat barbiturate poisoning. What is this compound called?**

Picrotoxin.

❍   **In the mid 1990s, there was seen the use of an Asian *"mushroom tea"* which was supposedly a fountain of youth. The substance was actually a symbiotic yeast-and-bacterial aggregate surrounded by a permeable membrane. Supposedly linked to possible liver toxicity, what was this product commonly called?**

"Kombucha," "Manchurian Tea," or *"Kargasok Tea."*

❍   **What plant did the physician Avicennia, consider the most fatal to humans of all poisons?**

Hellebore.

❍   **The Anglo-Saxons called it *"thung"* a word which became synonymous with any poisonous plant, and the Greeks called it *"lycotonum."* What poisonous plant were they describing?**

Aconite, *Aconitum napellus.*

❍   **Pliny reported the use of this plant in 1400 BC by a soothsayer and physician named *Malampus*. Because of this association, this toxic plant is sometimes referred to as *"Melampode."* What plant was so described?**

Black Hellebore, *Helleborus niger.*

❍   **The common name of this toxic plant comes from the Anglo-Saxon words for *"shore"* and *"a plant,"* and the scientific name is derived from the Greek word *"konas"* to *"whirl about,"* as intoxication caused vertigo. What plant was so described?**

Hemlock = *"hem"* (shore) + *"leac"* (a plant), *Conium maculatum.*

❍   **The early writer Albertus Magnus attributed the effects of this toxic plant to the planet Jupiter, and named it *"Acharonis."* The dead in *Hades* were supposedly crowned with the same plant. And the ghost in *Hamlet* was murdered with it. What plant was so described?**

Black Henbane, *Hyoscyamus niger.*

❍   **It is a grass with poisonous seeds. Medieval peasants were sometimes poisoned when they failed to follow the Biblical warning to separate the weeds from the grain. What plant caused this problem?**

Tares, *Lolium temulentum.*

❍   **A tourist pamphlet to the Virgin Islands, warns visitors NOT to sit under this poisonous tree for fear of contact with the highly irritating sap, which the Indians once used to make poison arrows. What is the name of this plant?**

The "Manchineel Tree," *Hippomane mancinella.*

❍   **In 1828, the first U.S. ambassador to Mexico, brought back home a native plant that many believe to be poisonous, but it really poses little problem. What was the plant?**

"Poinsettia," by Dr. Joel Poinsett.

❍   **The plant *Jatropha curcas*, contains within its seeds *"Hell Oil,"* an oil more potent than Castor oil in causing purging. By what more common name is this plant known?**

"Barbados Nut."

❍   ***Asthmador*® cigarettes, once smoked by asthmatics, contained what toxic plant material?**

"Jimson Weed," *Datura stramonium.*

❍   ***"Dawamesk"* is a popular African green cake made from sugar, spices, orange juice, and the tops of what psychoactive plant?**

Cannabis.

❍   **In January 1997, Sam Sebastiani, Jr., of the California wine-making family died after consuming what type of wild mushroom?**

"The Death Cap," *Amanita phalloides.*

❍   **This toxic plant is usually found on the Thanksgiving holiday table as a decoration. The common name is actually an oxymoron. What is the plant's common name?**

"Bittersweet."

❍   **In 1900, in order to reduce public skepticism that this fruit might be poisonous, a Stillwater, Oklahoma, grocer had students from *Oklahoma A&M* eat some before a camera. What relatively newly introduced fruit was being promoted?**

Bananas.

○ **Eating the seeds of what plant, used in culinary creations, can result in a false positive test for opiates in the consumer?**

Poppy seeds.

SPORTS

○ **Which baseball *Hall of Famers*, were known as *"Big Poison"* and *"Little Poison"*?**

Paul and Loyd Warner.

○ **In September 1994, the world lost a prominent sports figure. Who's death from carbon monoxide poisoning shocked the tennis world?**

Vitas Gerulaitis.

○ **What famous baseball pitcher's career was severely curtailed by pulmonary exposure to poisonous gas during World War I?**

Kristi Mathewson.

○ **Soccer madness spreads throughout the world whenever the *"World Cup"* is played. Which country has fans so wild for their team that their word for fans is *"tifosi"* which means *"carriers of typhoid"*?**

Italy.

○ **Of all the sports teams in the *NFL*, *CFL*, *NHL*, *NBA*, *AL*, and *NL*, what are the only teams that are named after venomous animals?**

The Charlotte *"Hornets,"* and the Arizona *"Diamondbacks"* (Phoenix).

○ **Before being released, he served 8 years of a 122 year sentence in San Quentin, for the murder of his tenth wife. His end came in 1940 when this punch-drunk former world middleweight and welterweight boxer committed suicide by swallowing a bottle of sleeping pills in his sleazy Detroit hotel room. What was the name of this down and out sports figure?**

Norman Selby, *aka "Kid McCoy."*

○ **In the early days of baseball, some pitchers used to color the ball with the juice of a toxic plant, to darken it and make it harder for the batter to see. What plant material did they use?**

Tobacco juice.

○ **The abuse of cocaine, is felt to have contributed to the sudden death of what basketball star, on June 19, 1986?**

Len Bias.

❍ On January 5, 1975, an *"All-star"* baseball player with the *Houston Astros* committed suicide by means of carbon monoxide. Who was he?

Don Wilson.

❍ On March 28, 1907, the manager of the *Boston Red Sox*, Chick Stahl committed suicide, with what toxic agent?

Phenol, "carbolic acid."

❍ The worst season record in major league baseball history, 20 wins and 134 losses, was set in 1899, by a Cleveland team with the name of a venomous critter. What was the team's name?

The Cleveland *"Spiders."*

❍ You are watching a *NCAA* basketball game between Richmond and Georgia Tech. What two venomous creatures are represented by the team names?

"The Spiders" (Richmond) *vs. "The Yellow Jackets"* (Georgia Tech).

❍ In the game of baseball, they called me *"Cobra"* because of the speed of my bat. I was an all-star outfielder for the *Pittsburgh Pirates* and the *National League's Most Valuable Player* for 1978. What is my name?

Dave Parker.

❍ The year was 1904, and the Olympics were taking place in St. Louis, Missouri, with American, Thomas Hicks, competing in an event. It was significant because this was the first known case of performance-enhancing drug use in the Olympic Games, when his supporters plied him with brandy and strychnine (used in small quantities as a stimulant. In what event was he competing?

The *Marathon*.

❍ On May 10, 1963, what pro football player died of a suspected heroin overdose?

Eugene *"Big Daddy"* Lipscomb.

❍ *New York Yankee* pitcher David Cone once said, *"If we lose this game, I'm ready to go for the cyanide tablet."* Who had the *Yankees* just played?

The *"New York Mets."*

❍ What is the venomous nickname of the Arizona baseball team?

"The Diamondbacks."

❍   A special mixture of sand and clay was sent to Russia from Sweden to cover a clay court for a *Davis Cup* tennis match. Why did the material have to be sent back?

Because it was radioactive, having seven times the normal emission.

❍   The sport of baseball, often has giveaway days. In 2000, the *Colorado Rockies* gave away key chains which were blamed for causing what type of poisoning in a toddler?

Lead.

❍   On September 19, 1896, *"Cannonball"* Crane, the famous pitcher for the New York *"Giants,"* died from an overdose of what drug substance?

Chloral hydrate.

SUBSTANCES

○ Because of its ability to cause rapid unconsciousness, what toxic gaseous compound is sometimes known as *"knockdown gas"*?

Hydrogen sulfide, or H_2S.

○ To the nearest %, what part of the weight of the compound Ferrous sulfate is represented by elemental iron?

20% *w/w*.

○ A familiar poem goes: *"Poor little Tommy, with us he is no more, for what he thought was H$_2$O was H$_2$SO$_4$."* What is H_2SO_4?

Sulfuric acid.

○ Made by altering the solubility of the alkaloidal salt from a member of the genus *Erythroxylon*, and precipitating it from an aqueous solution to produce irregularly shaped pieces of hard solid material, this commonly abused substance has taken on the common street name of what?

"Crack" or *"Rock."*

○ What toxic compound is produced when one mixes bleach with ammonia?

Chloramine gas.

○ This chemical once used as a rodenticide, can cause hair loss as a classic toxicological manifestation. What is the chemical?

Thallium.

○ The condition known as *"Orange-Picker's Flu"* is caused by low-level chronic exposure to what?

Organophosphate pesticides.

○ The odor of *"pears"* on the breath is a clue to the presence of what drug in the victim?

Chloral hydrate.

○ This odorless, tasteless, and colorless compound results from the incomplete combustion of fossil fuels. What is the chemical name of this toxic gas?

Carbon monoxide, or CO.

O   **Ingestion of this particular acid may cause a dermal rash which has sometimes been called the *"Boiled Lobster Syndrome."* What is the name of this acid?**

Boric acid.

O   **Why would contact with *CN*, *CR*, or *CS*, not be a laughing matter?**

They are all crowd control lacrimators.

O   **If you got a good whiff of $CHCl_3$, would you be most apt to: make a date with a beauty queen, take a nap, or run for the nearest exit?**

Take a nap, as it is Chloroform.

O   **A condition commonly known as *"blackjack disease,"* is characterized by non-ulcerative eczematous dermatitis, and is found in card players who are in prolonged contact with the green felt on card tables. What toxic metallic substance in the material causes this condition?**

Chromium.

O   **The trade name of what carbamate insecticide sounds like a cardinal number?**

Sevin®, generically named Carbaryl.

O   **Which word in the following series does NOT belong: *MDA*, *PCP*, *ASA*, *THC*?**

ASA, which is the acronym for aspirin (Acetyl salicylic acid). All the other are acronyms for different drugs of abuse.

O   **An unpleasant and potentially toxic condition results when particles of amorphous carbon and tarry substances, the product of incomplete combustion, form the nuclei of fine condensation of vapor over a considerable area. What do we call this condition?**

Smog.

O   **List the four major vitamins which are fat soluble?**

A, *D*, *E*, and *K*.

O   **What chemical can be synthesized in the laboratory, but occurs naturally in the mineral *"Sassolite,"* and is used as an herbicide, an insecticide, a flame retardant, and an antiseptic?**

Boric acid.

❍ **Which word in the following toxic series does NOT belong: kerosene, gasoline, turpentine, naphtha?**

Turpentine. The others are hydrocarbon fractions from crude oil, while turpentine comes from pine trees.

❍ **Drinking in a sleazy bar in New Orleans in 1890, a man was robbed after someone slipped him a *"Mickey Finn."* What chemical had been placed in his drink?**

Chloral hydrate.

❍ **The Family name of the ant lead to the naming of an organic acid which was first isolated by distillation of ant bodies. What is the name of this acid?**

Formic acid, from family Formicidae.

❍ **What commercial product, manufactured by the firms *Tesch/Stabenow* and *Degesch*, has killed more people than any other product in history, resulting in the deaths of hundreds of thousands of victims?**

Zyklon B (or *Cyclone B*), used in the German death camps during *World War II*.

❍ **If an employee of a chemical laboratory said he had just been accidentally exposed to a combination of *Unnilhexium*, *Unnilpentium*, and *Unillquadium*, what substances would he be talking about?**

The newest of the chemical elements, #s 104-106, *Unh*, *Unp*, and *Unq*.

❍ **What is the more colorful name of the antidote potassium ferricyanoferrate?**

"Prussian Blue."

❍ **Arsine is to arsenic as what is to antimony?**

Stibine.

❍ **What important antidote is isolated from the fungus *Streptomyces pilosus*?**

Deferoxamine.

❍ **In 1990, a Florida resident died from drinking a bottle of a nonalcoholic-beer drink named *"Pony Malta de Bavaria."* What had the product been contaminated with that caused his demise?**

Cocaine, as 37-54 grams had been added in Columbia, for smuggling purposes.

❍ **The average internal surface area, in square *meters*, found in a single *gram* of normal activated charcoal, is: 10, 100, or 1,000?**

$1,000 \ m^{2.}$

O   *Naloxone* is to codeine, as what is to *diazepam*?

The pure antagonist *Flumazenil*, or *Mazicon*® by Roche.

O   **The *Cyanide Antidote Package* manufactured by *Pasadena* (formerly *Lilly*), consists of three different chemicals. What are they, in the order in which they are normally administered?**

Amyl nitrite - Sodium nitrite - Sodium thiosulphate.

O   **The year 1930, saw the introduction of a Lithium containing drink called "*Bib-Label Lithiated Lemon-Lime Soda,*" which was touted to relive the depression caused by hangovers. Still on the market, but without the Lithium, what is this popular drink now called?**

7-Up®.

O   **On February 10, 1894, what important antidote class was claimed to have been discovered by the team of Phisalix and Calmette?**

Antivenin.

O   **We know that lead glaze in dinnerware can be toxic, but when one mixes tin and lead (4:1), one gets a metal widely used in Colonial days to make dinnerware. What was this substance called?**

Pewter.

O   **In 1994, it was reported that to get high, some Persian Gulf adolescents in Dubai, in the Emirate of Abu Dhabi, were smoking, or inhaling the fumes from the crushed material, of something called "*Samaseem.*" Paying up to $135 for a small packet, what unusual material makes up this intoxicating substance?**

Ants.

O   **What *Schedule I* drug, now subject to abuse, was openly offered to visitors at the Turkish booth at the 1876 *Centennial Exposition* in Chicago, Illinois?**

Hashish.

O   **It isn't really poison, but is a perfume by that name. Who manufactures this fragrant product?**

Christian Dior.

O   **Methylchloroform chloro acetophenone is sometimes found in a woman's handbag and when confronted can cause a rather nasty experience. By what more common name is this product known?**

Mace®, from the chemical name Methylchloroform chloroACEtophenone.

○   **What toxic gas can be found in mines, where it is called *"stink damp"*?**

Hydrogen sulfide, or H_2S.

○   **The *"Lee-Jones Test,"* which yields a blue-green color, is proposed as a quick bedside test for what toxic chemical?**

Cyanide.

○   **When exposed to water or weak acids, the rodenticide zinc phosphide releases what toxic compound?**

Phosphine gas.

○   **What symptoms are included in the classic "diagnostic triad" for *PCP*?**

Nystagmus, hypertension, and fluctuating levels of consciousness.

○   **What drug, sold and used primarily in Europe and Japan, is a derivative of the *Rauwolfia* plant, and which has been reputed by the Poison Center in Paris, France, to result in a 24% fatality rate, in overdoses?**

Ajmaline, or *Gilurytmal*.

○   **How was the association first made between alcohol consumption and the potential toxic effects of the drug Disulfiram?**

In the 1930s, when employees of rubber plants stopped at bars on the way home, and suffered strange symptoms. They had been working with the industrial chemical sulfiram, in treating rubber.

○   **In France, on March 16, 1915, the manufacture and consumption of a potent alcoholic liquor distilled from wine and wormwood, became illegal. What was the name of this toxic drink which was popular with French artists of the period?**

Absinthe.

○   **This drug was first introduced in the 1950s in India and Africa as a antimalarial. By 1972 it had become the 6th best selling sedative/hypnotic, and in 1973 was classified as a *Schedule II* drug because of its abuse potential. It became popular with the drug culture who mixed it with alcohol. What drug was this?**

Methaqualone, or *Quaalude*®.

○   **Since this group of drug chemicals was discovered in 1863 by the Belgian, Aldolph von Baeyer, on the *Feast Day of Saint Barbara*, he combined the Saint's name and the chemical name *"urea,"* to name what group of now abused substances?**

Barbiturates,

❍   **First introduced in 1862, it remains the oldest prescription sleeping medication available today. When mixed with ethanol, it becomes a thing popular in detective fiction. What is the name of this substance?**

Chloral hydrate,

❍   **This pesticide used against potato beetles, corn pests, and rape plant parasites, was banned by the *EPA* in the United States in 1974. It is also known by the trade names: *Compound 497*, *HEOD*, and *Octalox*. By what generic name is it known?**

Dieldrin,

❍   **This volatile oil has been used by some persons in attempted abortions. It has a name which sounds like a high class type of money. What is it?**

Pennyroyal Oil.

❍   **This poison was popular throughout Europe in the 1400s, and was made by feeding arsenic to toads and then distilling the juices from their dead bodies. By what name was this poison known to the peoples of the day?**

"Venin de crapaud."

❍   **To bind 9 *milligrams* of elemental iron, one would require how many *milligrams* of Deferoxamine: 10, 100, 500, or 1,000?**

100 *mg.*

❍   **In the body, Methylene chloride can be converted to what toxic compound?**

Carbon monoxide.

❍   **The ingestion of what potent herbicide, precludes treatment by the administration of oxygen?**

Paraquat.

❍   **This decay product of *Radium-226,* has now become an environmental concern as a cause of lung cancer. What is the name of this potential domestic hazard?**

Radon gas.

❍   **In 1968, Paul Krassner, editor of the *Realist*, threatened to add what to Chicago's water supply, in order to disrupt the national Democratic Convention being held in that city?**

LSD.

❍   **In 1966, the Sandoz company turned over all its supplies of what drug to the** *National Institute of Mental Health*?

LSD.

❍   **What was the trade name of the** *OTC* **product (containing Sodium bicarbonate, with tartaric and citric acids), who's advertisers claimed it to be the** *"antidote for intestinal toxicity"*?

Eno®.

❍   **Near Hidalgo, Texas, in October 1990, a new toxic immigrant entered the United States. Who or what was it?**

The arrival of the *Africanized* or *"Killer Bees."*

❍   **In 1836, James Marsh published his method for the detection of what toxic substance?**

Arsenic.

❍   **There has been discussions of late, regarding the addition of a bitter aversive agent to toxic products to reduce the likelihood of large ingestions. What is the name of this substance?**

Denatonium benzoate, or *Bitrex*®.

❍   **The English** *Royal Society of Physicians* **officially issued lists of medicines to be carried by London pharmacies. What poison antidote was finally dropped from the list in 1746?**

"Unicorn" horn.

❍   **Basil Valentine, a Benedictine monk living in the 15**th **Century, carried out experiments by giving small amounts of a toxic metal to his brother monks, recording his results in a work titled** *"Triumphal Chariot of* [blank]*."* **What toxic metal's name would complete the title?**

Antimony.

❍   **Which member of the following group of substances would NOT be expected to cause** *bullous lesions*: **carbon monoxide, snake venom, acetaminophen, barbiturates, or methaqalone?**

Acetaminophen.

❍   **What drug has been described as having the smallest therapeutic/toxic ratio of any commonly used medication?**

Digitalis.

❍   **What do the following items have in common toxicologically: candles, crayons, rouge, mascara, and artist's chalk?**

They are all considered nontoxic in normal exposure amounts.

❍   **The *"Ferric Chloride Test,"* which turns urine blue or violet, is a test for what group of compounds?**

Phenolic compounds.

❍   **Name the toxic cyclic polymer chemical which can be used as a cloud seeding chemical, an anesthetic, a fuel, or a slug/snail bait.**

Metaldehyde.

❍   **When washing skylights, it was common practice in England, in the early 1900s, to add a teacupful of what toxic chemical to a bucket of water to prepare the cleaning solution?**

Hydrofluoric acid (60% concentration).

❍   **Approximately what percent of the some 60,000 chemicals used in science have been tested for toxic effects: 10%, 30%, or 50%?**

30%.

❍   **First written about in the year 1140 AD, their name is said to be from the Persian *"pad-zahr"* (*"an expeller of poison"*). By what more familiar name do we know these folklore antidotal objects?**

Bezoars.

❍   **In 1874, the *Boston Medical Surgical Journal*, reported the first incident in English of lead poisoning from what source?**

A retained bullet.

❍   **What is the most lethal man-made chemical, being 150,000 times as potent as cyanide, with an *LD* of $3.1 \times 10^{(-9)}$ moles/kg?**

TCDD, or 2,3,7,8-tetrachlorodibenzo-*p*-dioxin (3 ounces could kill the population of New York City!).

❍   **The viable spores of the microorganism *Bacillus thuringiensis* have found a commercial use as what?**

An insecticide.

○   **Introduced into Eastern medicine by the Arabs, this antidote which consisted of growths in the intestines of animals, made when calcareous materials accumulated around a foreign body, are better known as what?**

Bezoar stones.

○   **In the *"Reinsch Test"* for arsenic, what common nonmetallic chemical can result in a false positive test by plating out on the copper?**

Sulfide.

○   **What substance is commonly added to many airplane and model cements in order to discourage solvent abusers?**

Oil of mustard, chemically known as allyl isothiocyanate.

○   **In 1858, the Belgian physician Sovet described symptoms among three servants who had been polishing silver with a white powder. Their symptoms included vomiting, stomach cramps, abdominal pain, sore throat, and tightness in the chest. These were the first recorded cases of poisoning by the carbonate of what toxic metal?**

Cadmium.

○   **Which word in the following series does NOT belong: Magnesium sulfate, Magnesium citrate, Sodium sulfate, Sodium chloride?**

Sodium chloride. All the others can be utilized in toxicology as laxative agents.

○   **What commonly abused substance is chemically named 1-hydroxyethane?**

Ethanol.

○   **Ingestion of aged cheeses, yeast products, beer, wine, citrus fruits, broad beans, snails, chicken liver, or pickled herring, can produce a classic toxic food/drug interaction which what group of medications.**

MAO Inhibitors.

○   **A mothball which has a wet and shiny appearance is most likely to contain what chemical?**

Paradichlorobenzene.

○   **We all know that botulism toxin is very potent, but in 1990, the *FDA* approved the use of *Oculinum*® (an injectable form of *Type A* botulism toxin) for the treatment of what medical conditions?**

The eye muscle disorders: *strabismus* and *blepharospasm*.

○   **The lightest weight element which is a solid, is a toxic metal. What is it?**

Lithium.

○   **This substance was used liberally by the alchemist Paracelsus, and he carried it in the pommel of his saddle referring to it as the *"stone of immortality."* It is also possible that the famous Arab physician Avicenna may have died of a self-administered overdose of this substance. Its active ingredient was named by Serturner after the Greek god of sleep. What is this substance?**

Opium, or Morphine.

○   **In the 1830s, a patent medicine was sold under the name of *"Dr. Miles' Compound Extract of Tomato."* It is NOT considered toxic and is still around today by what better known generic name?**

Ketchup.

○   **We have often herd of vitamins like *B₁* and *B₆*, but what is *Vitamin B₁₇*?**

Laetrile, the cyanogenic glycoside.

○   **What are the names of the two major active alkaloidal compounds which are found in Syrup of Ipecac?**

Emetine and Cephaeline.

○   **Of the two types of phosphorus, red or yellow, which type ignites on contact with air?**

Yellow.

○   **What toxic substance produces a peanut-like odor on the breath?**

Vacor, a rat poison.

○   **What chemical is no longer used in the routine bathing of newborn babies because of its ability to cause neurological disorders?**

Hexachloraphene.

○   **The famous Italian sculptor and goldsmith Benvenuto Cellini (1500-1571), described in his biography of being poisoned by the fumes of what toxic metal?**

Mercury.

○   **Many organophosphate insecticides have a characteristic of what odor?**

Garlic.

❍   A common street drug combination is *"Ts and Blues."* What two drugs make up this combination?

T = Pentazocine/Talwin®, *Blues* = Tripelenamine/Pyribenzamine®.

❍   The odor of *"violets"* on the breath is a clue to the presence of what substance in the victim?

Turpentine.

❍   What is the generic name of the veterinary drug *Sernylan*® which has found an abuse potential on the street?

Phencyclidine.

❍   The Aztecs called it *"teonanacatl"* (God's flesh), and used it in their religious ceremonies, but what kind of material was this?

Mushrooms, usually members of genus *Psilocybe.*

❍   Which of the following drugs, would NOT be expected to cause opiate like symptoms: pentazocine, diphenoxylate, oxazepam, or propoxyphene.

Oxazepam, a benzodiazepine drug.

❍   To the nearest whole %, what is the concentration of Sodium hypochlorite in most standard liquid household bleaches?

5% *w/v.*

❍   What is probably the most widely used of all mind altering drugs. Being commonly ingested in food, beverages, or proprietary medications?

Caffeine.

❍   A high-school student was found in a supermarket, sniffing the foaming agent from aerosol cans of whipped cream. What common anesthetic substance was being abused?

Nitrous oxide.

❍   A Mexican folk remedy for the treatment of *"empacho"* (caused by a blockage of the digestive tract), utilizes common substances which in Spanish are called *"greta"* and *"azarcon."* What is the toxic constituent of these substances than can lead to severe problems?

Lead. *"greta"* = lead oxide, *"azarcon."* = lead tetraoxide.

❍   An antidote called *"silymarin"* obtained from the "Milk Thistle," *Silybum marianum*, is thought by some to be beneficial for intoxication by what toxic compounds?

Amatoxins, from mushrooms.

❍   When this alcohol is metabolized in the body it oxidizes to a toxic chemical more likely to be found in a funeral parlor. What is this alcohol called?

Methanol or *"Wood Alcohol."* The metabolite is formaldehyde.

❍   In its time *"Theriac"* was worth its weight in gold. What is *"Theriac"*?

A universal poison antidote consisting of over 61 ingredients, which became the most famous cure-all medicine ever known, being officially available from 70-1870 A.D.

❍   The first modern description of this metal's toxicity was the famous study by Tanquerel des Planches, in 1839, which was based upon 1,200 cases of poisoning. What was this metal?

Lead.

❍   What toxic cleaning compound found in many homes, was used by Chinese potters, as early as 600 BCE, to glaze their pottery?

Borax.

❍   In 1990, the illicit use of what substance by body builders, that caused *CNS* depression, lead to *FDA* bans and warnings?

GHB, gamma-hydroxy-butyrate.

❍   The ingestion of what rodenticide can produce the odor of rotten fish on the patient's breath?

Zinc phosphide.

❍   It's native sulfide was used by women in Egypt and in the East for darkening the eyebrows and eyelids. In the 16th and 17th centuries it was alloyed with tin to produce *"pocula emetica"* which were kept in monasteries so that monks who took too much wine could be punished by having to drink from these *"emetic cups"* (when filled with wine, the wine would become impregnated with tartar emetic). This toxic metal was known to the ancients as *"stibium"* or *"stimmi."* What is this toxic metal?

Antimony.

❍   Before it fell into disfavor, this substance was used to induce vomiting in medical facilities. What derivative of compounds from the *"Poppy"* was so used by injection?

Apomorphine.

❍   **The use of this metal's salt in the 1940s and 1950s, as a substitute for table salt led to intoxications and its withdrawal from the market. What was the name of this elemental metal?**

Lithium.

❍   **What antidote is the drug of first choice for reversing the effects of *"cholinergic overdrive"*?**

Atropine.

❍   **What toxic agent can cause luminescence of the vomitus and feces, and causes the *"smoking stool syndrome"*?**

Yellow phosphorus.

❍   **If you mix a white metal that burns violently in water with a yellowish-green poisonous gas, you get what edible substance?**

"Table Salt," sodium chloride, NaCl, (from sodium + chlorine).

❍   **On August 18, 1991, an Oshkosh, Wisconsin man ingested a tablet contaminated with strychnine, where upon he was stricken with seizures and hospitalized. What was the product he took?**

Spanish Fly Pills®, by Legendary Sex Exciter.

❍   **In 1985, a ship arrived in California, bearing a toxic cargo that caused quite an alarm amongst agriculturists. What was its unexpected cargo?**

"Killer Bees."

❍   **EMS or *"Eosinophilic-Myalgia-Syndrome"* has been associated with the use of what health food product?**

L-tryptophan.

❍   **In 1991, thousands of bottles of *"Agua Destilada"* (distilled water) were removed from pharmacy shelves in Puerto Rico and the Virgin Islands because, through a labeling error, the bottles actually contained what toxic product?**

Rubbing Alcohol, or Isopropanol.

❍   **Airbags in cars are becoming more standard in the industry. What is currently the principal chemical explosive component and major potential toxin?**

Sodium azide.

◯   An essay by physician William Heberden, in 1759, resulted in the elimination of what long time accepted poison antidotes from the *London Pharmacopoeia*, in 1788?

Theriac and *Mithridate*.

◯   This rodenticide compound was first found in the South African plant called "gifblaar" (*Dichapetulum cymosum*). It is produced commercially under the trade name *"Compound 1080."* What is the chemical name of the toxic active ingredient?

Sodium monofluoroacetate.

◯   In 1991, testimony in a United States Senate hearing on Indian Affairs stated that the biggest problem on the reservations among today's Native American youth was the consumption of alcohol from what unlikely commercial product?

Lysol Disinfectant Spray, containing 79% *v/v* ethanol.

◯   What is the color of chlorine gas?

Greenish-yellow.

◯   Some individuals are allergic to dyes used in foods. Give the common name for the following *"FD&C"* dyes: (a) *Red No. 3*, (b) *Red No. 4*, (c) *Yellow No. 2*, (d) *Yellow No. 5*.

(a) Erythrosine, (b) Panceau, (c) Amaranth, (d) Tartrazine.

◯   Street fentanyl overdoses have caused fatalities and are often confused with heroin intoxication. Give the street name used for this substance on the East Coast and West Coast.

East Coast = *"Tango and Cash,"* West Coast = *"China White."*

◯   List the four ingredients from which activated charcoal is made?

Burnt wood, coconut, bone, and sucrose, or rice starch.

◯   Indicate which more common odor is often associated with each of the following substances: (a) butyl nitrate, (b) phenol, (c) nystatin, (d) carbon disulfide, (e) zinc phosphide.

(a) Dirty socks, (b) white paste, (c) cereal, (d) rotting cabbage, (e) raw liver.

◯   If one takes forwards the letters or combination of letters in the word *IPECAC*, one will find the atomic symbols for five different elements of the Periodic Table. Name the elements, in order.

I = iodine, *P* = phosphorus, *Ca* = calcium, *Ac* = actinium, *C* = carbon.

○   One day a family enters a poison center with a box containing old chemical bottles found in the attic of a house they just purchased. The contents of the bottles are only identified with the names which were commonly used in days of old. What substance does each of the bottles contain if the names used are as follows: **(a)** *Aqua Fortis*, **(b)** *Aqua Potabilis*, **(c)** *Condy's Crystals*, **(d)** *Spirits of Salt*, **(e)** *Salt of Saturn.*

(a) Nitric acid, (b) Water, (c) Potassium permanganate, (d) Hydrochloric acid, (e) Lead acetate.

○   The odor of a toxic substance can often be associated with the odor of some more familiar substance one may have experienced. Given the toxic substance, give the common item that has often been listed as having a similar odor: **(a)** Aniline, **(b)** Coniine, **(c)** Vacor, **(d)** Amyl acetate, **(e)** Cicutoxin.

(a) Shoe polish, (b) Mouse urine, (c) Peanuts, (d) Bananas, (e) Carrots.

○   One day a family enters a poison center with a box containing old chemical bottles found in the attic of a house they just purchased. The contents of the bottles are only identified with the names which were commonly used in days of old. What substance does each of the bottles contain if the names used are as follows: **(a)** *Oil of Mirbane*, **(b)** *Oil of Cassia*, **(c)** *Chenopodium Oil*, **(d)** *Oil of Niobe*, **(e)** *Oil of Palma Christi.*

(a) Nitrobenzene, (b) Cinnamon oil, (c) American Wormseed oil, (d) Methyl benzoate, (e) Castor oil.

○   **What is considered to be the most poisonous *natural* substance known to man?**

Botulinus toxin, LD_{50} = 500 nanograms.

○   **Here are some questions concerning the use in the USA of the antidote N-acetylcysteine (*NAC*) to treat Acetaminophen overdose. Answer the following: (a) What is the loading dose, (b) What is the maintenance dose, (c) How many total doses are to be administered, (d) For oral administration, it should be diluted to what final concentration?**

(a) 140 *mg/kg*, (b) 70 *mg/kg*, (c) 18 doses, (d) 5%.

○   **Arrange the following hydrocarbons in order by their viscosity (highest viscosity to lowest): gasoline, mineral seal oil, lubricating oil.**

Lubricating oil (>100 *SSU*) > Gasoline (<60 *SSU*) > Mineral Seal Oil (35 *SSU*).

○   **Answer the following about botulism: (a) Where does the word botulism originate, (b) What is the scientific name of the microorganism which produces the toxin, (c) Which Type of *botulinus* toxin is usually associated with contamination of fish and marine life?**

(a) From the Latin word *"botulus"* for sausage, (b) *Clostridium botulinum*, (c) *"Type E."*

❍   Here are three clues to the identity of a toxic substance. FIRST CLUE: It was prepared originally in the 1960s as a derivative of the opium alkaloid thebaine. SECOND CLUE: It is used on dart tips for the immobilization of large zoo animals. THIRD CLUE: It is listed in the *Guinness Book of World Records*, as the most powerful analgesic known, where even needle scratches can cause coma, and the human lethal dose is in the range of 30-120 micrograms.

Etorphine hydrochloride, *Immobilon*, or *M99*.

❍   Here are three clues to the identity of an historical drug. FIRST CLUE: While serving as a nurse during the *"War Between the States,"* author Louisa May Alcott (author of *Little Women*) was poisoned while being treated for *"TB,"* with this medication. SECOND CLUE: William A. Hammond, Surgeon General during the American Civil War, was removed from his post in May, 1863, for ordering the removal of this laxative drug from field hospitals. THIRD CLUE: When physicians in the Union Army flooded Washington, D.C., with demands to remove the Surgeon General, it became known as the *"[blank] Rebellion."*

Calomel, or Mercurous chloride.

❍   One day a family enters a poison center with a box containing old chemical bottles found in the attic of a house they just purchased. The contents of the bottles are only identified with the names which were commonly used in days of old. What substance does each of the bottles contain if the names used are as follows: (a) *Lunar Caustic*, (b) *Hasting's Naphtha*, (c) *Quicklime*, (d) *Spirits of Hartshorn*, (e) *Paris Green*?

(a) Silver nitrate, (b) Methanol, (c) Calcium oxide, (d) Ammonium hydroxide, aqueous, (e) Copper acetoarsenite.

❍   One day a family enters a poison center with a box containing old chemical bottles found in the attic of a house they just purchased. The contents of the bottles are only identified with the names which were commonly used in days of old. What substance does each of the bottles contain if the names used are as follows: (a) *Prussic Acid*, (b) *Acid of Sugar*, (c) *Oil of Vitriol*, (d) *Potash*, (e) *Quicksilver*?

(a) Hydrogen cyanide, (b) Oxalic acid, (c) Sulfuric acid, (d) Potassium carbonate, (e) Mercury.

❍   Here are three clues to the identity of a poison. FIRST CLUE: Darwin published an account of the use of *Upas Tieute* for the execution of criminals in the Malay Peninsula. SECOND CLUE: It has been described as one of the most bitter substances known, with a taste detectable at a dilution of 1:700,000. THIRD CLUE: The seeds, which come from a tree, containing the poison are sometimes called *"Poison Nuts."*

Strychnine.

O   State whether the following pesticides are used to combat rodents, insects, or plants: **(a) Paraquat, (b) Brodifacoum, (c) Agent Orange, (d) Thallium, (e) Pyrethrin.**

(a) Plants, (b) Rodents, (c) Plants, (d) Rodents, (e) Insects.

O   **In the 1980s, a case was made by the ethnobotanist, Wade Davis, for the main ingredient of voodoo powders used in Haiti to produce zombification. What did he conclude was the main active component of these *"Zombi Powders"*?**

Tetrodotoxin.

O   **Name the organism which causes the type of food poisoning that has plagued the dairy industry over the last few years, leading to recalls of contaminated cheese and ice cream.**

Listeria monocytogenes.

O   **What would each of the following agents be used to treat: (a) Thioctic acid, (b) Hydroxocobolamin (Vit. B$_{12a}$), (c) Fuller's Earth, (d) *BAPN*, (e) Calcium gluconate gel, (f) *Prussian Blue*.**

(a) Amatoxins, (b) Cyanide, (c) Paraquat, (d) Corrosives/caustics, (e) Hydrofluoric acid, (f) Thallium.

O   **Here are three clues to the identity of a famous toxic agent. FIRST CLUE: It was responsible for the Middle Age malady known as *"St. Anthony's Fire."* SECOND CLUE: It comes from the invasion of cereal crops by the organism *Claviceps purpurea*. THIRD CLUE: It finds use in modern medicine in the treatment of migraine headaches.**

Ergot, or Ergotamine.

O   **Name the three common ingredients found in the older recipe for *"Universal Antidote."***

Burnt toast, strong tea, and Milk of Magnesia.

O   **State whether the following fumes are lighter or heavier than air: (a) Carbon monoxide, (b) Methane, (c) Hydrogen cyanide, (d) Ammonia, (e) Chlorine.**

(a) Lighter, (b) Lighter, (c) Lighter, (d) Lighter, (e) Heavier.

O   **And now to test you knowledge of the use of poisons in capital punishment in the United States. Answer each of the following: (a) On February 28, 1924, the poisonous gas Hydrogen cyanide was first used to execute a criminal, of Chinese origin, who was convicted of a gang-style killing. What was the name of the gas chamber's first victim, (b) In what state did the first execution by gas take place, (c) On December 6, 1982, Charles Brooks, was the first criminal to be executed by**

"lethal injection." In what state did this execution take place? (d) What three different chemicals or drugs were used in the lethal injection process?

(a) Gee Jon, (b) Nevada, (c) Texas, (d) Sodium thiopental, Pancuronium bromide, and Potassium chloride.

◯   **Combinations of street drugs sometimes have very unusual names. Indicate what chemicals or drugs are found in each of the following street named combinations: (a) *"Black Dust,"* (b) *"Dynamite,"* (c) *"Fours and dor's,"* (d) *"Killer Weed,"* (e) *"OJ,"* (f) *"R and R."***

(a) *PCP* + Heroin + Emblaming fluid, (b) Marijuana + Heroin, (c) Codeine + Glutethimide (Doriden), (d) Marijuana + *PCP*, (e) Opium + Marijuana, (f) Seconal + Ripple wine.

◯   **Indicate what drug or group of drugs each of the following acronyms stand for: (a) *NSAID*, (b) *TCA*, (c) *MAOI*, (d) *INH*, (e) *DBI*.**

(a) Nonsteroidal antiinflammatory drugs, (b) Tricyclic antidepressants, (c) Monoamine oxidase inhibitors, (d) Isoniazid, (e) Phenformin.

◯   **What plant growth regulator was subsequently withdrawn from the market in 1989, after it came under public attack in the 1980s for its cancer causing potential, as a residue on apples?**

Alar, Diaminozide.

◯   **They come in many toxic varieties including: *"tulip," "striated," "textile,"* and *"geographer."* What are they?**

Cone shells.

◯   **In the olden days mistakes were sometimes made when *Ipecac Fluid Extract* was used in place of *Ipecac Syrup*. How many times more potent is the *Fluid Extract* than the *Syrup*?**

14 times.

◯   **In olden days, *"Gosio gas"* was commonly found in rooms with a musty smell. What was felt to be the source of this toxic compound?**

Moldy wallpaper, which generated Trimethylarsine gas.

◯   **Before being changed by international convention, in 1903, a homicidal poisoner could easily obtain very toxic Phosphorus from what common source around the home?**

Matches.

○   For centuries the Chinese have used *"Ch'an Su,"* the dried venom of what common animal for external application as a medicinal agent?

The toad.

○   What antidote against an anticoagulant is obtained from the sperm of fish?

Protamine.

○   What anticoagulant is obtained from a snake called *Bothrops atrox moojeni*?

Batroxobin.

○   In the 1980s a new form of Mexican heroin began to appear in North America. Because of its color and consistency to a roofing compound, it was commonly called by what name?

"Black Tar" heroin.

○   The toxic compound styrene was first discovered in 1827, and there is only one known naturally occurring styrene product? What is it?

Organic acids of *Storax balsam*.

○   When used medicinally in France, the drug *Stalinon*, was found to case severe neurological sequellae, with more than 100 deaths. What compound was the cause?

Diethyl tin, and/or Triethyl tin.

○   The first antivenin for treating snakebite was produced in 1895, at what world famous biological institute?

Pasteur Institute, Paris, France.

○   What medicinal plant substance is also known as *"vegetable arsenic"*?

Colchicine.

○   In 1925, oily suspensions of this substance were used to treat syphilis, and severe poisonings resulted before the proper dose could be determined. What was the elemental cause of these iatrogenic poisonings?

Bismuth.

○   In the 1800s, a popular drink called *"Vin Mariani,"* was even given an official seal of approval by Pope Leo *XIII*. It did however, contain a plant product which is now prohibited. What was it?

Cocaine.

○   Oscar Wilde said of this toxic drink *"After the first glass you see things as you wish they were. After the second, you see things as they are not. Finally you see things as they really are, and that is the most horrible thing in the world."* What liquid in the glass was he describing?

Absinthe, containing toxic *thujone* from *"Wormwood."*

○   One of the first polyatomic molecules discovered in interstellar space, was a toxic compound. What was it?

Cyanide.

○   In 1639, Woodal, described a particular substance as follows: *"It is the hottest, the coldest, a true healer, a wicked murderer, a precious medicine and a deadly poison."* What toxic material was he describing?

Mercury.

○   In 1993, scientists were able to synthesize the compound *epibatidine*, a powerful non-opiate analgesic. This compound is a normal component of the venom of what toxic creature?

Arrow-poison frogs.

○   In the 1800s, many individuals became addicted to this product the name of which comes from the Latin *"something to be praised."* By what more common name is it known?

Laudanum, or Tincture of Opium.

○   In 1930, 15 milligrams of a substance was first isolated from 25,000 liters of policemen's urine, which today has lead to abuse by macho individuals to obtain rapid results with minimal pain. What is this specific substance called?

The anabolic steroid *"Androsterone."*

○   *Benzpril, Captopril,* and *Enalapril,* are examples of compounds known as *ACE* inhibitors. What does the acronym *ACE* stand for?

Angiotensin-Converting-Enzyme

○   In 1994, it was reported that the drug *Flunitrazepam* was being abused in Europe, Asia, and South America. Legally available as *Rohipnol* in other countries, what slang is used by abusers, for this drug?

"Roofies."

○   In 1995, there was reported a new designer drug from Germany, which was a small gray tablet marked with a triangular-headed cartoon character. Chemically similar to *"Ecstacy"* (*MDMA*), what is the common name of this drug?

"Fido Dido."

○ **In the Far East, a toxic substance was known as *"pen yen."* What addictive toxic substance is so called?**

Opium.

○ **This substance found to be 20-25 times more potent than the naturally occurring Tetrodotoxin or Batrachotoxin, is found in the *Palythoa* or soft corals of the Caribbean and Pacific oceans. What is this very toxic compound called?**

Palytoxin, or *PTX.*

○ **What is *"Vitamin Q"*?**

The slang term for Methaqalone.

○ **In POISINDEX® one will find a listing for a substance known as *"Obecalp."* Is it considered toxic, and what is it?**

Nontoxic. It is *"Placebo"* spelled backwards!

○ **During 1995, in New York City, four men died from ingesting a supposed aphrodisiac. It was a brown, rock-like substance containing toad secretions. By what common name was it sold in specialty shops?**

"Stone," or *"Black Stone,"* or *"LoveStone."*

○ **Thomas Lewis Lavy hanged himself in jail after being arrested for attempting to bring 130 grams of a toxic substance from Alaska into Canada. What was this substance, which is believed to be the third most deadly, exceeded only by Plutonium and *Botulinus* toxin?**

Ricin.

○ **Imported from Thailand, this product, often in the form of a powder ball, and known as *"Choua Zoua Nea,"* is popular among immigrant South East Asians for the purposes of cleaning. It has also proven a popular suicidal agent. What is the exact use and toxic agent of this product?**

Silver cleaner, containing Cyanide.

○ **This early antidote was made by macerating musk, aristolchia (probably *Aristolochia longa* or *A. clematis*), *"Birthwort,"* and scorpions, together in wine. It was given a common name associated with a famous early queen. What was the name of this magic antidote?**

"Confection of Cleopatra."

❍   **In 1996, there was approved the drug *Bentoquatam* 5%. What was innovative about this substance?**

Known as *"Ivyblock,"* it was the first drug approved to protect against Poison Ivy.

❍   **For many years, the *OTC* product *"APC,"* was a popular analgesic. But one of the components was judged to be too harmful, and it fell into disuse. What was the toxic component?**

Phenacetin.

❍   **In 1970, the *FDA* banned the use of home dry-cleaning products which contained what toxic chemical substance?**

Carbon tetrachloride.

❍   **Shortly after 1948, the British medical journal *Lancet*, urged that British detectives stop using *"gray powder"* for fingerprint development, due to toxicological complications experienced by law enforcement personnel. What was the toxic component of this investigational tool?**

It contained 33% Mercury.

❍   **Known to the ancients, this toxic alkaline gaseous compound was called *"vehement odor"* by Pliny. What is the chemical name of this dangerous compound?**

Ammonia.

❍   **This heavier than air gaseous compound was also known as *"death gas,"* *"creeping killer,"* or *"invisible death."* What is the chemical name of this dangerous compound?**

Carbon dioxide.

❍   **In 1812, the scientist Charles Waterton, made a journey into *Dutch Guiana*, to learn about a specific botanical poison. What was he in search of?**

Curare.

❍   **In India and nearby regions, a product known as *"Surma"* is commonly used, which may be toxic containing 26-83% lead. For what purpose is it used?**

Eye makeup.

❍   **In 1665, in Indrija, Yugoslavia, this substance became the first to be the cause of legislation to control its occupational disease. What was the substance?**

Mercury.

○   **In 1295, Marco Polo reported** *"hoof rot"* **disease in horses in the mountains of Turkestan, from the ingestion of grass from soil which was rich in what element?**

Selenium.

○   **What drug was considered the first apparent transplacental carcinogen in humans, causing cancer of the genital tract in female offspring?**

Diethylstilbestrol, *DES*.

○   **What toxic substance was often referred to as** *"magical mineral,"* **supposedly being used by the** *Vestal Virgins* **for the wicks of their oil lamps?**

Asbestos.

○   **In 1939, the Swiss chemist Paul Mueller discovered the insecticidal properties of what chemical, which was to have a great impact on the world's ecology?**

DDT.

○   **What toxic gas used in World War I, had the faint smell of musty hay or green corn?**

Phosgene, or Carbonyl chloride.

○   **During the** *"American Centennial Exposition"* **of 1876, many Philadelphia pharmacies openly sold what substance of abuse?**

Hashish.

○   **What chemical is used in** *"nontoxic"* **antifreeze?**

Propylene glycol.

○   **In 1984, 23 Baltic Sea fishermen were poisoned when a container broke open they had accidentally hauled up from the deep. What chemical was released upon them when the artillery shells ruptured?**

Mustard Gas.

○   **The year 1869 saw the development of the first synthetic sedative hypnotic drug. What was it?**

Chloral hydrate.

○   **The 1969 case of** *California vs. Woody*, **established the Constitutional right to consume what controlled drug in the religious ceremonies of a specific church?**

Peyote.

○   Once ipecac was mixed with 10% opium to produce a drug used to induce sweating to treat fever. What was this preparation called?

"Dover's Powders."

○   Among one of the top 50 chemicals produced in the USA, it is used as a gasoline additive as well as to dissolve cholesterol gallstones. It is called *MTBE*. What does this acronym stand for?

Methyl-*tert*-Butyl Ether.

○   In June 1997, Karen Wetterhahn, a Dartmouth College cancer research scientist, died from the effects of a relatively rare heavy metal compound which had passed through her latex rubber gloves ten months earlier. What very toxic mercurial compound, first synthesized in 1841, she was studying?

Dimethyl-mercury.

○   What is the formulation relationship between the modern aperitifs *"Pernod"* and *"Ricard,"* and the once toxic drink *"Absinthe"*?

They have the same formulation, without the *Wormwood*.

○   In ancient Colombia, some nursing mothers practiced infanticide by smearing their nipples with extracts from what plant species?

Datura.

○   In 1934, Dr. Mary Walker first used what chemical substance, a poison antidote to treat patients with *Myasthenia gravis*, which came to be known as *"the miracle of St. Alpheges"*?

Physostigmine.

○   What unusual toxic substance has been known to be ingested by some cocaine abusers in an attempt to prolong the drug's effects by reducing its metabolism?

Organophosphates.

○   In 1915, the first U.S. drug manufactured in tablet form was produced. It became popular with the public, yet was very toxic in high doses. What was the drug?

Aspirin.

○   In 1938, a new toxic substance was synthesized, which was subsequently named after it's developers: Schrader, Ambrose, Rudringer, and Vander Linde. What acronym was used for the name?

Sarin.

○ **In 1952, while searching for a new pesticide to replace *DDT*, Dr. Ranajit Ghosh, synthesized what very toxic compound?**

"VX" nerve gas.

○ **The compounds of Arsenic can have various colors associated with their common names. What color is associated with each of the following forms of arsenic: (a) Arsenic disulfide, (b) Beta arsenic, (c) Arsenic trisulfide. (d) Arsenic trioxide.**

(a) Red, (b) Black, (c) Yellow, (d) White.

○ **Place the following four toxic agents in order, by their LD$_{50}$, from lowest to highest: Strychnine sulfate, Morphine sulfate, Tetrodotoxin, and Nicotine.**

Morphine - Strychnine - Nicotine – Tetrodotoxin.

○ **Many people get into dermal trouble when coming into contact with chiles. According to their *Scoville* units for capsaicin effect, list the following chiles in order from mildest to hottest: *"Puya," "Ancho," "Pasilla," "Habanero,"* and *"Pequin."***

"Ancho" (1,000), *"Pasilla"* (2,500), *"Puya"* (5,000), *"Pequin"* (75,000), *"Habanero"* (300,000).

○ **If one were working in waterfront dive on the Barbary Coast of San Francisco, during the late 1800s, one would have to know how to concoct some of the drugging potions used to shanghai or rob certain bar patrons. Supply the correct recipe for each of the following popular concoctions: (a) *"Miss Piggot Special,"* (b) *"Shanghai Smoke"*?**

(a) Equal parts gin + whisky + brandy, laced with laudanum, (b) A cigar laced with opium.

○ **Many metallic substances can be toxic, but do you know what metals can be found in different mineral substances? Give the major metallic substance in each of the following minerals: (a) Pyrite, (b) Galena, (c) Halite, (d) Chalcocite, (e) Cinnabar?**

(a) Iron, (b) Lead, (c) Sodium, (d) Copper, (e) Mercury.

○ **In 1965, the *FDA* changed from prescription to *OTC* status, what important poisoning treatment item?**

Syrup of Ipecac.

○ **Some toxic substances can have a color mentioned in their common name. Give the color found in the common name of each of the following: (a) *Agriope aurantia*, (b) *Caulophyllum thalictroides*, (c) *Loxosceles reclusa*, (d) *Urginea maritima*, (e) *Dendroaspis viridis*.**

(a) *"Golden"* Orb-weaver spider, (b) *"Blue"* Cohosh, (c) *"Brown"* Recluse spider, (d) *"Red"* Squill, (e) *"Green"* Mamba.

O   **Some toxic substances can have a color mentioned in their common name. Give the color found in the common name of each of the following: (a)** *Pseudonaja textilis,* **(b)** *Latrodectus mactans,* **(c)** *Crotalus scutulatus scutulatus,* **(d)** *Vespula pennsylvania,* **(e)** *Robina pseudoacacia.*

(a) *"Brown"* Snake, (b) *"Black"* Widow spider, (c) Mojave *"Green"* Rattlesnake, (d) *"Yellow"* Jacket, (e) *"Black"* Locust.

O   **One day a family enters the poison center with a box containing old chemical bottles found in the attic of a house they just purchased. The contents of the bottles are only identified with the names which were commonly used in days of old. What substance does each of the bottles contain if the names used are as follows: (a) Photogen, (b) Camphene, (c) Daturine, (d) Wood naptha, (e) Coal naptha.**

(a) Kerosene, (b) Turpentine, (c) Atropine, (d) Methanol, (e) Benzene.

O   **What toxic substance has sometimes been called the** *"great imitator"* **because of the range of symptoms that have been described in its intoxication?**

Carbon monoxide.

O   **How many types of** *botulinus* **toxins have been described?**

7 (*"A"* through *"G"*).

O   **One day a family enters a poison center with a box containing old chemical bottles found in the attic of a house they just purchased. The contents of the bottles are only identified with the names which were commonly used in days of old. What substance does each of the bottles contain if the names used are as follows: (a)** *Blue Oil,* **(b)** *Carbon Oil,* **(c)** *Columbian Spirit,* **(d)** *Gum Oil,* **(e)** *Fastitious Air?*

(a) Aniline, (b) Benzene, (c) Methanol, (d) Oil of Turpentine, (e) Nitrous oxide.

O   **One day a family enters a poison center w/ith a box containing old chemical bottles found in the attic of a house they just purchased. The contents of the bottles are only identified with the names which were commonly used in days of old. What substance does each of the bottles contain if the names used are as follows: (a)** *Ague Tree Oil,* **(b)** *Floras Martis,* **(c)** *Cologne Spirits,* **(d)** *Dutch Oil,* **(e)** *Gas Black?*

(a) Sassafras Oil, (b) Ferric chloride, (c) Ethanol, (d) Ethylene dichloride, (e) Carbon Black.

O   **The scientist Karl Wilhelm Scheele isolated the poison Prussic Acid by adding Sulphuric acid to what substance used as an antidote for a heavy metal?**

"Prussian Blue."

○   During the *Middle Ages*, what material, now known to be non-toxic, was considered to be the most poisonous substance?

Diamond.

○   One day a family enters a poison center with a box containing old chemical bottles found in the attic of a house they just purchased. The contents of the bottles are only identified with the names which were commonly used in days of old. What substance does each of the bottles contain if the names used are as follows: (a) *Glauber's Salt*, (b) *White Precipitate*, (c) *Checkerberry Oil*, (d) *Dakin's Solution*, and (e) *Cyanogas*?

(a) Sodium sulfate, (b) Ammoniated Mercuric chloride, (c) Wintergreen Oil, (d) Sodium hypochlorite in water, (e) Calcium cyanide.

○   One day a family enters a poison center with a box containing old chemical bottles found in the attic of a house they just purchased. The contents of the bottles are only identified with the names which were commonly used in days of old. What substance does each of the bottles contain if the names used are as follows (a) *Plumbago*, (b) *Saltpeter*, (c) *Cucumber Dust*, (d) *Vinegar Naptha*, and (e) *Monsel's Salt*?

(a) Graphite, (b) Sodium or Potassium nitrite, (c) Calcium arsenate, (d) Ethyl acetate, (e) Ferric subsulfate.

○   What common baking ingredient did the U.S. Air Force use to replace more toxic paint strippers?

Sodium bicarbonate, *"Baking Soda."*

○   What spice substance is usually forbidden in prisons, as it can be used as a weapon when thrown in the eyes?

Black Pepper.

WORDS

○ The unit of measuring the viscosity of a petroleum hydrocarbon is the *"SSU."* For what do the letters *SSU* stand?

Saybolt Seconds Universal.

○ The last name of what prominent clinical toxicologist rhymes with the name of a plant which can caus allergic skin reactions?

"Rumack" (Barry), which rhymes with *"Sumac"* (Poison).

○ If you were a psychotherapist, and one of your patients complained to you of having *"iophobia,"* what sort of problem would he have?

The fear of being poisoned. From the Greek *ios* ("poison") + *phobia* ("abnormal fear").

○ In 1970, the establishment of the *PPPA* provided a great step forward in reducing accidental exposures to poisons in children. What is the *PPPA*?

Poison Prevention Packaging Act.

○ In 1852, the English chemist Robert Angus Smith wrote a 600 page book about this subject, and created a term that is very much in the environmental headlines today. What is the term?

"Acid rain."

○ What word do we use in toxicology which comes from the Greek words for *"against"* plus *"to give"*?

"Antidote." From the Greek *anti-* + *didonai*.

○ The Japanese ideograph for what animal that can bite as well as sting, is a composite of the characters for *insect, unselfishness, justice,* and *courtesy*?

The ant.

○ According to slang in the British Royal Navy, what food is referred to as *"poison on armor plate"*?

Ship's biscuits dipped in beef tea.

○ What four letter word is a slang term for: cocaine, deceptive talk, and interference on one's *TV*?

"Snow."

❍   **The name of what group of antidotes, comes from the Greek word for the large claw of a lobster or crab?**

Chelators.   From the Greek *"chela."*

❍   **Sometimes a single word can have opposite meanings. What word of Greek origin means *"remedy"* as well as *"poison."***

"pharmakon."

❍   **A mnemonic device for remembering those drugs which may be radiopaque is the acronym *CHIP*. What do these letters stand for?**

Chloral hydrate - Iron – Phenothiazines.

❍   **The word *"toadeater"* has come to mean a person who flatters others for self-serving reasons. How did the word originate?**

A *toadeater* was a charlatan's assistant, who pretended to eat a toad so his employer could display his ability in expelling the poison.

❍   **Just to be different, here is a question to test your ability to work in another language, and so is delivered in French. *Vrai ou faux? Les feuillages de pomme de terre, sont bonne pour manger?***

Faux! The leaves of the potato are NOT good to eat, they are toxic.

❍   **Most people in toxicology are aware of the unusual condition of poisoning called "[blank] *Syndrome By Proxy*." Correctly spell the name of the Syndrome.**

M-u-n-c-h-a-u-s-e-n

❍   **What French word is spelled almost like poison, does NOT mean poison, but can be a vector for poison?**

"Poisson," the word for fish.

❍   **Where did we ever get the name *"heroin"* for the drug Diacetylmorphine?**

It is the trade name registered by the *Bayer Company* for the drug product which they developed and marketed in the late 1800s.

❍   **Only a single letter separates the spelling of two sound-alike toxic substances. One is the simplest of the aromatic compounds, and the other is a commercially prepared mixture of aliphatic and aromatic hydrocarbons. Spell them, and tell which is which.**

Benzene = single ring aromatic, and *Benzine* = the aromatic mixture.

○ **We all know that a *nanogram* (one billionth of a gram) represents a very small amount of a poison. But where did the prefix *"nano"* originate?**

From the Greek *nanos*, a dwarf or *"little old man."*

○ **Its name was derived from the Latin word for sugar, and it was used as a sweetening agent until its ban by the *FDA* in 1977. What is it?**

Saccharin.

○ **In recent years there has been a lot of environmental concern of the toxic effects from *UFFI*. What do these letters stand for?**

Urea Formaldehyde Foam Insulation.

○ **Where did the acronym for the hallucinogenic chemical *"LSD"* originate?**

From the German *Lyserge Saure Diethylamid.*

○ **In the diagnosis of lead poisoning, one hears the terms *ALA* and *EP*. To what do these terms refer?**

ALA = delta-aminolevulinic acid, *EP* = erythocyte protoporphyrin.

○ **A child drinks from a container which is labeled *"VM and P Naphtha."* For what do the letters *VM and P* stand?**

"Varnish Maker's and Painters" Naphtha.

○ **The *Chemical Manufacturers Association* operates *CHEMTREC*, established to provide information during chemical emergencies. For what do the letters *CHEMTREC* stand?**

CHEMical TRansportation Emergency Center.

○ **In the future, intoxicated patients will probably be treated with specifically designed *"Fab" fragments*, like the currently produced *Digibind*®. For what do the letters *FAB* stand?**

Fragments Antigenic Binding.

○ **The *FDA* maintains a list of chemicals used in foods which is commonly known as the *GRAS* (pronounced "grass") list. For what do these letters stand?**

Generally-Recognized-As-Safe.

○ **What is the term for the production of abnormalities in developing organisms during uterine life?**

Teratogenesis.

❍   **What Federal legislation having to do with hazardous materials and the community's right-to-know, sounds like a girl's first name?**

"SARA," the Superfund Amendments and Reauthorization Act.

❍   **The name antimony is thought to have originated from the French word *"anti-moine."* What did this mean in French?**

"hostile to monks."

❍   **The word used to describe the first milk taken from a cow after birthing a calf, sounds like the words used to describe the results of handling some *Apis mellifera*. What is the word?**

"Beestings."

❍   **What term is used to describe the immunity from poison that is realized after taking a series of small doses?**

"Mithridatism."

❍   **In marijuana the active ingredient is known as *THC*. For what do the letters *THC* stand?**

Tetrahydrocannabinol.

❍   **In assessing the dangers of atmospheric intoxications, the term *IDLH* is often used. For what does this acronym stand?**

Immediately Dangerous to Life and Health.

❍   **What is the drug world's slang term for a cigar which has been gutted, and has had the tobacco replaced with marijuana?**

"Blunt."

❍   **BHT is an antioxidant commercially used as a food preservative. What do the letters *BHT* stand for?**

Butylated hydroxytoluene.

❍   **We have all heard of Puccini's opera *"La Tosca,"* but what does the acronym *TOSCA* stand for in toxicological legislation?**

Toxic Substances Control Act, of 1976.

❍   **The collecting of wild mushrooms for food is common to many countries and cultures. Spell the word for *"mushroom"* in each of the following languages: (a) French, (b) German, (c) Spanish, (d) Latin.**

(a) *Champignon*, (b) *Pilz*, (c) *Hongo*, (d) *Fungus*.

❍   **Tell what drug the following acronyms stand for: (a) *HCTZ*, (b) *LSD*, (c) *MDA* , (d) *PZI*, (e) *PPA*.**

(a) Hydrochlorothiazide, (b) Lysergic acid diethylamide, (c) Methylenedioxyamphetamine, (d) Protamine zinc insulin, (e) Phenylpropanolamine

❍   **Give the more complete name for each of the following toxicologically related laboratory tests: (a) ALA, (b) *G6PD*, (c) *PTT*, (d) *SGOT*, (e) *SGPT*.**

(a) delta-aminolevulinic acid, (b) Glucose-6-phosphate dehydrogenase, (c) Partial Thromboplastin Time, (d) Serum Glutamic-Oxaloacetic Transaminase, (e) Serum Glutamic-Pyruvic Transaminase.

❍   **Many common maxims in English are associated with a toxic naturally occurring animal. Complete each of the following common phrases: (a) *a ...in the grass*, (b) *a ...in the bosom*, (c) *a ...of deceit*, (d) *a ...tongue*.**

(a) *snake*, (b) *viper*, (c) *web*, (d) *waspish*.

❍   **In the world of analytical toxicology, indicate for what each of the following instrumental acronyms stand: (a) *HPLC*, (b) *TLC*, (c) *GC*, (d) *MS*, (e) *IR*, (f) *AA*.**

(a) High-pressure Liquid Chromatography, (b) Thin-layer Chromatography, (c) Gas Chromatography, (d) Mass Spectrophotometry, (e) Infrared Spectrophotometry, (f) Atomic Absorption Spectrophotometry.

❍   **We have all heard the words ending in *-cide*, from the Latin *"caedere"* (to kill). Words like pesticide and suicide. Who, or what, would be the intended poison victim in each of the following types of killings: (a) *matricide*, (b) *avicide*, (c) *uxoricide*, (d) *felicide*, (e) *senicide*.**

(a) a mother, (b) a bird, (c) a wife, (d) a cat, (e) the elderly.

❍   **Many countries have snakes. Spell the word for *"snake"* in the following languages: (a) German, (b) French, (c) Spanish, (d) Italian, (e) Japanese.**

(a) Schlange, (b) Serpent, (c) Serpiente, (d) Serpente, (e) Hebi.

❍   **We have all heard the words ending in *-cide*, from the Latin *"caedere"* (to kill). Words like pesticide and suicide. Who or what would be the intended poison victim in each of the following types of killings: (a) *genocide*, (b) *vaticide*, (c) *patricide*, (d) *avunculocide*.**

(a) a race, (b) a prophet, (c) a father, (d) an uncle.

❍   **You are about to travel through Asia, stopping in the cities of Jerusalem, Damascus, Bombay, Beijing, Hanoi, and Manila, and would like to talk to the people about poisons in their locations. What is the word for *"poison"* in each of the** following native languages: **(a) Hebrew, (b) Arabic, (c) Hindi, (d) Mandarin, (e) Vietnamese, (f) Tagalog.**

(a) *"Sam,"* (b) *"Sim,"* (c) *"Zehar"* [pronounced *"za-hair"*], (d) *"Dew,"* (e) *"Chat doc"* [pronounced *"jock dow"*], (f) *"Lason"* [pronounced *"lah-son"*].

○   **Indicate the words which each of the following acronyms stand for in the area of industrial toxicology: (a) *TLV*, (b) *PEL*, (c) *IARC*, (d) *TWA*, (e) *STEL*.**

(a) Threshold Limit Value, (b) Permissible Exposure Limit, (c) International Agency for Research on Cancer, (d) Time Weighted Average, (e) Short-term Exposure Limit.

○   **Define the following words which incorporate the prefix *"tox-"*: (a) *Toxicide*, (b) *Toxicophidia*, (c) *Toxicomania*, (d) *Toxicotabellae*, (e) *Toxopexic*.**

(a) A drug capable of overcoming toxic agents, (b) Venomous snakes, collectively, (c) An intense desire for poisons, (d) Poison tablets, (e) Making a poison harmless to an organism.

○   **Spell the word for *"poison"* in each of the following languages: (a) French, (b) Spanish, (c) German.**

(a) *Poison*, (b) *Veneno*, (c) *Gift*.

○   **For what do the following antidotal acronyms stand: (a) *BAL*, (b) *EDTA*, (c) *NAC*, (d) *HBO*.**

(a) British Anti-Lewisite, (b) Ethylene diamine-tetra-acetic acid, (c) N-acetylcysteine, (d) Hyperberic oxygen

○   **To the ancient Greeks what did the word *"pharmacopeus"* mean?**

A poisoner, or purveyor of toxic substances.

○   **During the Roman period, what did the word *"alexipharmic"* mean?**

Complex medicines that were considered to have antidotal properties against poisons in general.

○   **In 1837, Cantani in Italy, coined a term used to describe the toxic effects from eating plants such as *"Chick Peas."* What was this term?**

"Lathyrism."

○   **What term was coined in 1894, by the Italian physician L. Montano, to designate an acute hemolytic anemia following the ingestion of broad beans?**

"Favism."

❍   **What word sounds both like a toxic plant, and an article in the home to help people sleep by keeping out bothersome illumination?**

"Nightshade."

❍   **Envenomation from the *Hymenoptera* cause more deaths in the *USA* each year, than any other type of venomous animal. What is the derivation of the world *"hymenoptera"*?**

Hymen ("membrane") + *pteron* ("wing").

❍   **We all know that a drop of acid can be corrosive, but if a British mother said her child had an *"acid drop"* in his mouth what would she mean?**

It is a sour ball candy.

❍   **In Chinese Communist political terminology, what is meant by the words *"poisonous weeds"*?**

Any writings or allied propaganda which attacks Mao Zedong.

❍   **In the late 1800s in France, what did the French refer to as *"l'heure verte,"* that had a toxic connection?**

The *"green hour,"* of absinthe cocktails.

❍   **We all know that it is illegal to possess the active ingredients of the coca plant, but if you visit France, you can walk into many establishments and order *"Coca."* What will you be given?**

Coca Cola®.

NOTES

NOTES

NOTES

NOTES

NOTES